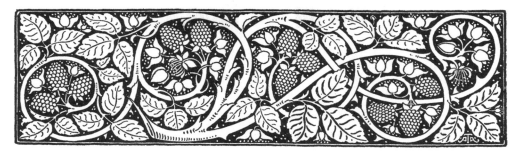

You can view this as a recipe book and use it as such, but I hope this book will inspire you to walk the path of the Hearth Witch, which is so much more. While you may begin to learn how to work with natural resources from books like this one, the true teaching only comes when you start listening to the land and its plants and animals.

When the sacred within you recognises the sacred that surrounds you everywhere, a deeper spiritual reality opens up in which all space becomes sacred space, all time becomes sacred time, and all acts become sacred acts.

This is the true path of the Hearth Witch. Walk it in beauty.

Anna Franklin

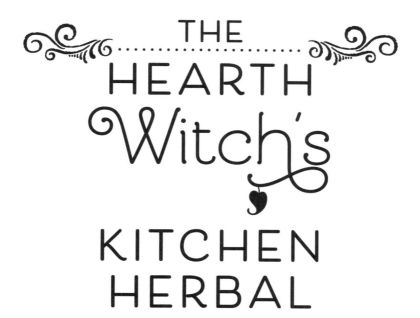

THE
HEARTH
Witch's
KITCHEN
HERBAL

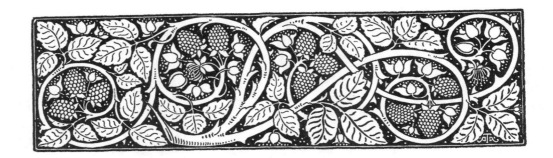

Anna Franklin is a third-degree witch and high priestess of the Hearth of Arianrhod, and she has been a practicing Pagan for more than forty years. She is the author of thirty books and the creator of the *Sacred Circle Tarot, Fairy Ring Oracle,* and the *Pagan Ways Tarot* (Schiffer, 2015). Her books have been translated into nine languages.

Anna has contributed hundreds of articles to Pagan magazines and has appeared on radio and TV. She lives and works in a village in the English Midlands, where she grows her own herbs, fruit, and vegetables, and generally lives the Pagan life. Visit her online at www.AnnaFranklin.co.uk.

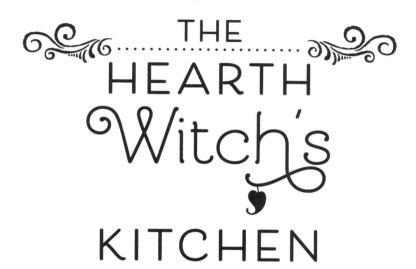

THE
HEARTH
Witch's
KITCHEN
HERBAL

CULINARY HERBS FOR MAGIC, BEAUTY, AND HEALTH

ANNA FRANKLIN

Llewellyn Publications
WOODBURY, MINNESOTA

FIRST EDITION
Second Printing, 2021

Book design by Rebecca Zins
Cover design by Shira Atakpu
Interior floral woodcut © 1167 Decorative Cuts (New York: Dover Publications, 2007)
Llewellyn is a registered trademark of Llewellyn Worldwide Ltd.

NOTE: The information in this book is provided for educational
and entertainment purposes only. It does not constitute
a recommendation for use.

Library of Congress Cataloging-in-Publication Data
Names: Franklin, Anna, author.
Title: The hearth witch's year : rituals, recipes & remedies through the seasons / Anna Franklin.
Description: First edition. | Woodbury, Minnesota : Llewellyn Publications, [2020] | Includes bibliographical references and index. | Summary: "*The Hearth Witch's Year* examines how the natural tides of the year shape the hearth witch's spiritual life, looking at how nature influenced spiritual practice in the ancient Pagan world and how it should influence us today, because when we are separated from nature, we are separated from our spiritual source. It includes seasonal rituals, practices, and recipes for every month of the year"—Provided by publisher.
Identifiers: LCCN 2020038124 (print) | LCCN 2020038125 (ebook) | ISBN 9780738764979 (paperback) | ISBN 9780738765174 (ebook)
Subjects: LCSH: Witchcraft. | Year—Religious aspects—Paganism.
Classification: LCC BF1566 .F6955 2020 (print) | LCC BF1566 (ebook) | DDC 203/.3—dc23
LC record available at https://lccn.loc.gov/2020038124
LC ebook record available at https://lccn.loc.gov/2020038125

Llewellyn Publications
A Division of Llewellyn Worldwide Ltd.
2143 Wooddale Drive
Woodbury MN 55125-2989

www.llewellyn.com
Printed in the United States of America

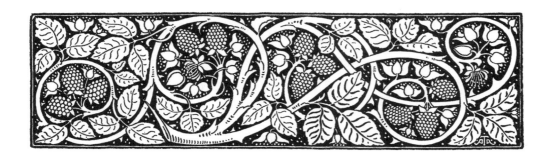

Contents

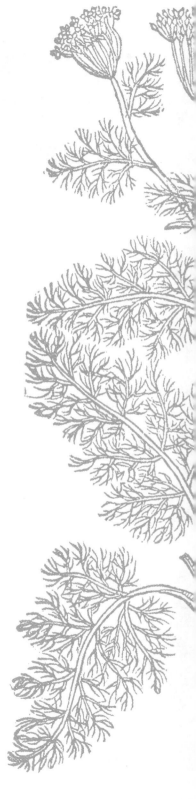

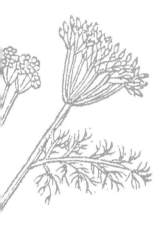

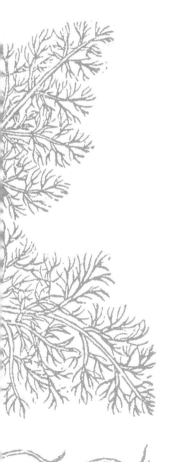

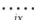

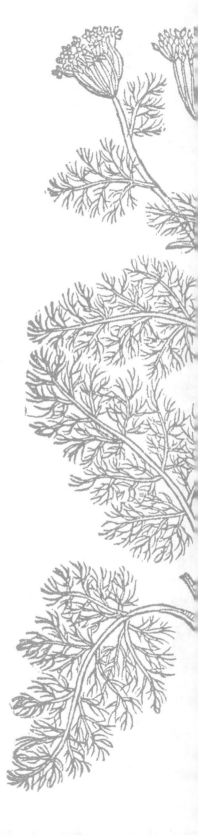

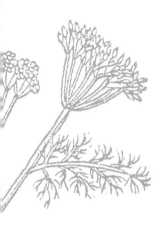

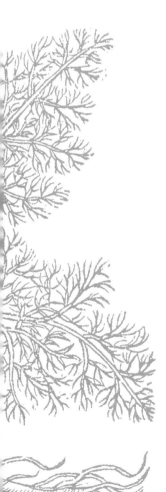

OTHER KITCHEN HERBS IN BRIEF

223

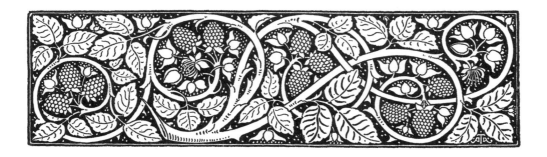

Introduction

• • • • •

The *Hearth Witch's Kitchen Herbal* is a herbal with a difference: it looks at the herbs and spices most of us already have in our kitchens and shows how they can be used for home remedies, personal care, spiritual practice, and magic.

I often visit Pagan conferences, markets, and camps, where I meet people looking around for the hottest trend or the latest magical or healing ingredient, and the rarer and more expensive it is, the more magical and useful they think it must be. This is nothing new. The spices we use daily for cooking were once extremely costly and rare, coming from faraway, exotic places, and because of this people scrabbled to get hold of them, believing they had mystical properties and greater healing powers than the herbs that grew at home—and sometimes this was true. It is hard to imagine now, but the black pepper you sprinkle on your dinner every evening was once one of the most valuable commodities in the world, worth its weight in gold because of its medicinal properties and culinary piquancy. When Christopher Columbus set sail on his voyage of exploration, it was to find a new route to get black pepper cheaper, but he landed in the New World and found chilli peppers instead. Other spices were so mysterious, they were thought to have magical origins. Cinnamon was believed to grow in deep glens guarded by deadly snakes, where the legendary phoenix birds built nests from it, immolating themselves so that they might emerge reborn from its ashes.[1] Naturally, this story justified the exorbitant prices that traders charged for it.

For our ancestors, plants were a wonderful treasure trove of natural resources that could be employed for food and medicine or be used to provide clothing, furniture, and building materials. However, it was also believed that they had a spiritual quality, and their employment in magic and religious practice was equally important.

Herbs and spices have been examined, tested, classified, and written about for millennia. Early herbals generally included the spiritual and magical aspects of plants as well as their uses in healing, and most of our knowledge on how our ancestors used plants comes from these. The earliest known herbals are the Chinese *Shennong Bencao Jing*, or "Great Herbal" (2700 BCE); the *Sushruta Samhita*, which documents the teachings of Ayurveda (traditional Indian medicine) and dates back to the second millennium BCE; and the Egyptian *Papyrus Ebers*, which dates to 1550 BCE but is believed to be based on sources two thousand years older. Several Greek and Roman herbals are still extant, and modern doctors still take the Hippocratic oath, which comes from the Greek herbalist Hippocrates (460–377 BCE), often called the father of medicine. Theophrastus (371–287 BCE), another Greek, founded the science of botany with his careful observations on plant growth, habitat, and distribution, documented in his *Historia Plantarum* and *De Causis Plantarum* ("On the Causes of Plants"). The *De Materia Medica* ("On Medical Materials"), written by the Roman army doctor Dioscorides around 65 CE, served as the model for herbals and pharmacopoeias for the next thousand years and was used right up to the Renaissance. A valuable resource on the ritual use of plants in the classical world is from Pliny the Elder (23–79 CE), whose comprehensive *Naturalis Historia* details plants, their medical uses, and their myths and legends.

The tradition of growing and using herbs in the west continued in the monastery gardens of Christian monks and nuns, who used their knowledge to heal themselves and the local community. One nun, the abbess Hildegard von Bingen (1098–1179 CE), became well known for her herbal healing ability, based on her study of classical texts and hands-on experience. She documented this in two books, *Physica* and *Causae et Curae*. When printing made books more affordable, the less wealthy could buy their own copies of herbals and make their own remedies. John Gerard's *Herball* of 1597 and *Culpeper's Complete Herbal* by Nicholas Culpeper (1653) are still in print.

---

1   Theophrastus, *Enquiry into Plants*.

How to Use This Book

In this book you will find guidance on making home remedies in your kitchen and learn how to prepare teas, tinctures, infused oils, electuaries, oxymels, and balms. There are also instructions on making and using personal care products for your face and hair, and some different ways of incorporating herbs into your magical and spiritual practice.

The A–Z kitchen herbal examines the most common herbs and spices that many of us have in our kitchen cabinets or grow in pots on the kitchen windowsill. This section documents their lore and their magical and spiritual virtues; as well, there are notes on their culinary and medicinal uses, with instructions on how to use them in home remedies, followed by some recipes for remedies, food, incense, cosmetic, and magical preparations. You will see how you can use something as simple as a herb tea for a variety of purposes, from healing to magic. Each of the sections will have any recipes that are to follow in bold type. Most of the recipes are very simple to prepare and use only one or two ingredients, but there are also more complex recipes if you want to delve further. This is intended to be an introduction to an art you can develop as you wish.

At the back of the book are some useful appendices on herbal terms, colours, and magical correspondences, plus quick reference guides to the cosmetic and medicinal uses of the herbs, other kitchen herbs in brief, and weights and measures.

A Note on Botanical Names

Many plants have similar names. The only way to be sure you have the right plant is to refer to the official botanical name, usually in Latin or Greek. This normally has two parts, the first referring to the genus the plant belongs to and the second referring to the specific species and usually descriptive, so that *Quercus rubra* translates as "oak red," with *quercus* meaning "oak" and *rubrus* meaning "red." The second part of the name can tell you a lot about the plant: *officinalis*, for example, means that it was a medicinal herb listed in the official pharmacopoeia, *vulgaris* means "common," *sylvestris* means "of the woods," *sativa* means "cultivated," and so on. Using botanical names isn't entirely foolproof as they are sometimes changed as the plants are reclassified and may appear differently in older books. Throughout this work I've tried to give both old and new botanical names. The older name will appear after the prefix *syn.*, meaning "synonym."

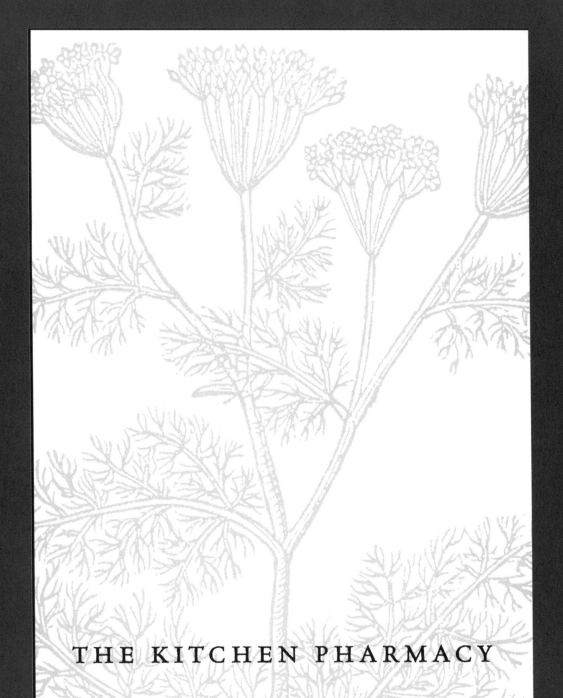

THE KITCHEN PHARMACY

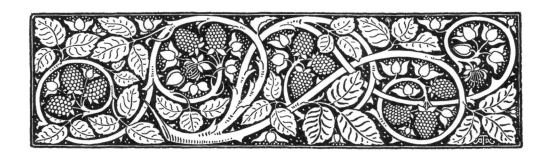

Making Your Own Herbal Remedies

· · · · · · ·

Your kitchen cupboard contains herbs and spices with valuable healing properties that can be used to treat and prevent common health problems. Most of us already use them in cooking, but they can also be thought of as friends that help us maintain wellbeing or treat common ailments. Using them can be as simple as incorporating them into your diet by making a cup of herbal tea.

Because we are using culinary herbs and spices, you can be sure that none of them are intrinsically harmful, but there are still a few safety considerations to be taken into account.

- Remember that anyone can be allergic to anything.

- Larger amounts of some herbs and spices are not compatible with prescription medicines. Always check with your healthcare professional before using herbal remedies on a regular basis.

- Always consult a medical practitioner if you have any acute or persistent health concerns.

- Make sure that you have looked up the method of preparation and the safe dosages.

- Do not take large amounts of any herb for an extended period of time.

Tools Needed

- Saucepan (not copper or aluminium)

- Double boiler (or a bowl over a pan of boiling water)

- Kettle

- Muslin

- Kitchen scales

- Measuring jug

- Bottles and jars

- Pestle and mortar

Herbal Preparations

Herbs may be prepared in a variety of ways for internal and external use, so let's look at some basic methods.

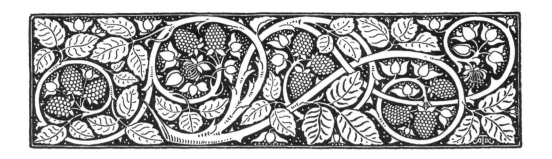

Internal Remedies

Infusions and Decoctions

Many of a herb's components, such as its minerals, vitamins, sugars, starches, hormones, tannins, volatile oils, and some alkaloids, dissolve well in water, and for this reason, herbs are often taken as infusions or teas (tisanes). Infusions can be made from the soft green and flowering parts of a herb.

A "strong infusion" indicates a greater measure of herbs to water. You can use a double-strength infusion to make a gargle for a sore throat, for example.

Some herbs have properties such as mucilage and bitter principles that are destroyed by heat, so a cold infusion is made.

Some of the harder, woodier parts of a plant, such as the seeds, roots, buds, and barks of our kitchen spices, need to be boiled in water for a while. This is called a decoction. If the herbs are dried, they should first be pounded into a powder.

Never use an aluminium or copper pan as those metals can react with the brew and taint it.

Herb Tea Basic Recipe

2 TEASPOONS FRESH OR 1 TEASPOON DRIED HERBS

250 MILLILITRES (1 CUP) WATER

Put the herbs in a teapot or a pot with a lid, pour on the boiling water, and infuse for ten to twenty minutes. Strain and sweeten with honey. Drink one to three times daily. A "double-strength" tea would mean using four teaspoons of fresh herbs or two teaspoons of dried herbs to 250 millilitres of water, doubling the quantity of herbs in the recipe.

Cold Infusion Basic Recipe

2 TEASPOONS FRESH OR 1 TEASPOON DRIED HERBS

250 MILLILITRES (1 CUP) WATER

Using a non-metal container, put in the herbs and water. Close the lid or cover with cling film (plastic wrap) and leave overnight. Strain before use. Take one to three times daily.

Decoction

2 TEASPOONS FRESH OR 1 TEASPOON DRIED HERB

250 MILLILITRES (1 CUP) WATER

Put the herbs in a pan and pour the water over them. Cover; if possible, let the herbs macerate in the cold water for a few hours. Put the pan on heat, bring to a boil, and simmer gently for fifteen to twenty minutes. Strain. Take one to three times daily.

Tinctures and Glycerites

These are fluid extracts of herbs using either alcohol or glycerine to extract plant chemicals and preserve them in an easily usable form that can be stored.

Plant constituents are generally more soluble in alcohol than water, and alcohol will dissolve and extract resins, oils, alkaloids, sugars, starches, and hormones, though it does not extract nutrients such as vitamins or minerals. A remedy made this way is called a tincture.

Brandy or vodka are usually used. Never use alcohols designed for external use, such as rubbing alcohol.

If you don't want to use alcohol for any reason or are formulating remedies for children, you can make a glycerite. I haven't included many glycerite recipes in the book, but be aware that you can use glycerine to extract phytochemicals from herbs in a similar manner to how alcohol is used to make a tincture, so you can convert the tincture recipes to glycerites. Vegetable glycerine can be purchased from pharmacies or online and is a syrup made from vegetable oil; it is very sweet but doesn't raise blood sugar, so it is safe for diabetics. Glycerine is a weaker solvent than alcohol, so glycerites won't be as potent as an alcohol-based tincture and you will need a larger dose for a therapeutic effect. They won't keep as long as a tincture and are not good at making extractions from hard barks and dried roots. Make sure you use a food-grade vegetable glycerine.

TINCTURE (FOLK METHOD)

To make a tincture, put 100 grams of dried herbs or 200 grams fresh herbs into a clean jar and pour on 500 millilitres of vodka or brandy. Seal and keep in a warm place for two to four weeks, shaking daily. Strain through muslin and store in a dark bottle in a cool place for up to two to six years. Because a tincture is much stronger than an infusion or decoction, you only need a few drops in a glass of water as a medicinal dose. Alternatively, a few drops may be added to a salve or bath.

GLYCERITE (FOLK METHOD)

To make a glycerite, put 100 grams of dried herbs or 200 grams fresh herbs into a clean jar and pour on 500 millilitres of slightly warmed glycerine. Seal and keep in a warm, dark place for two to four weeks, shaking daily. Strain through muslin and store in a dark bottle in a cool place for about a year. If you add water to your glycerite or use fresh herbs with a lot of water content, it will spoil much faster. Take a teaspoon three times daily.

Glycerine in itself is soothing for a sore throat. Glycerine is used in cosmetic products to soften, moisturise, and plump the skin, so you can use your herbal glycerites externally. Dilute with rose water to use as a skin toner or add to salves, creams, and soaps.

Syrups

Some herbs are bitter tasting and are more palatable when taken in the form of syrup, particularly for children. The sugar preserves the herbs. Thick syrup sticks to tissues, bringing the herbal benefits to sore throats and coughs.

SYRUP (FOLK METHOD)

To make syrup, first make your herbal infusion or decoction (see above), then for every 250 millilitres of infusion or decoction, add 250 grams of sugar and heat gently until the sugar is dissolved. Simmer gently until thickened. Pour into sterilised bottles and label. Unopened, this will keep six to twelve months in a cool, dark place. Once opened, keep in the fridge for one to two months. If you wish, you can use honey instead of sugar, though the heating process destroys most of honey's beneficial properties.

Herbal Vinegars

By just placing a few sprigs of herbs in vinegar, you can make herbal vinegars that are not only pleasant tasting when sprinkled on salads, but also therapeutic.

However, you can make a stronger version in the same way that you make a tincture, and this is an alternative to using alcohol. Though vinegar won't draw out as many phytochemicals from the herbs as alcohol, it does extract the vitamins and minerals from the plants. Acetas, or vinegar extractions, are not as strong as tinctures, so the dose needed is higher. Take two teaspoons three times a day. You can dilute your herbal vinegar with water to take internally, or use it externally in baths and compresses. Acetas generally have a cooling, anti-inflammatory effect, so are useful for conditions such as sore throats and inflamed skin. They will store for one to two years in a cool, dark place.

> Note: If you can, use raw cider vinegar.[2] Raw cider vinegar (the kind
> with the mother in it, rather than the barren pasteurised kind) contains
> antioxidants, vitamins and minerals such as magnesium and potassium, and
> helpful probiotic enzymes and bacteria. It stimulates digestion and has been
> shown to help lower blood pressure and increase HDL ("good") cholesterol.
> Though vinegar is acidic, cider vinegar has an alkaline effect on the body
> when consumed, which many people believe helps treat arthritis.

---

2   For an easy recipe to make your own raw cider vinegar, please see my *Hearth Witch's Compendium* (Llewellyn, 2017).

Electuaries (Herbal Honey)

An electuary is simply a herb or spice mixed with honey, so they are incredibly simple to make and will store for one to two years if dried herbs are used, or up to six months if fresh herbs are used (the water content from the fresh plant matter shortens the shelf life). Honey extracts both the water- and oil-based components from the herbs and is soothing and calming when added to a remedy. Take a teaspoonful one to four times a day.

Oxymels

Oxymels are a sweet and sour blend of honey and vinegar, combining the benefits of both. If you've ever taken apple cider vinegar and honey, you've had an oxymel. The easiest way to make a herbal oxymel is to mix an already prepared herbal electuary with a prepared herbal vinegar, generally a fifty-fifty mix. There are several oxymel recipes in this book, but you can come up with your own by simply combining different herb vinegars and electuaries, such as mixing sage electuary with rosemary vinegar, for example.

Another way to make an oxymel is to quarter fill a sterilised jar with dried herbs or half fill with fresh herbs and top up with a fifty-fifty mix of honey and slightly warmed vinegar. Put on a lid and keep in a cool, dark place, shaking daily. (Avoid using a metal lid, as this may be corroded by the vinegar and taint your product.) After two to four weeks, strain through muslin into a sterilised storage bottle.

For a quick way to make an oxymel, you can use the hot method. Simmer your herbs and vinegar together very gently, without boiling, for ten to twenty minutes. Strain out and stir in the honey while the vinegar is still warm.

The usual dosage of an oxymel is one to two teaspoons three or four times a day as needed (when you have a cold, for example). You can put a spoonful of oxymel in warm water and drink that, or even put a spoonful in a glass and top up with sparkling water or tonic water to create a herbal mocktail.

An oxymel should keep at least six to nine months in the fridge. Discard if you notice any mould.

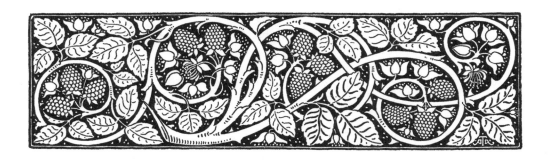

External Remedies

Baths

Adding herbs to a bath is a great way of getting the relaxing qualities of herbs (absorbed through the skin and inhaled) and for treating some skin conditions and aching muscles. You can put some herbs in a sock or muslin bag and drop this into the bath, but the bathwater isn't really hot enough to extract the herbs' qualities. The best way is to add 500 millilitres of herbal infusion or decoction (see page 10) to the bathwater and soak.

Steam Inhalations

Steam inhalations of herbs may be used to relieve cold symptoms (using peppermint, thyme, or ginger, for example).

STEAM INHALATION (BASIC METHOD)

1 LITRE BOILING WATER

2 TEASPOONS HERBS (FRESH, IF POSSIBLE)

Pour the boiling water over the herbs. With a towel over your head, inhale the vapour.

Salves

Herbs can be made into salves or ointments, which can then be applied to the affected area.

· · · · · · · · · · · · · · · ·
SALVES (FOLK METHOD 1)

200 GRAMS PETROLEUM JELLY

2 TABLESPOONS HERBS

In a double boiler, simmer the herbs in the petroleum jelly for twenty minutes. Strain into glass jars.

· · · · · · · · · · · · · · · ·
SALVES (FOLK METHOD 2)

250 MILLILITRES OIL

2 TABLESPOONS HERBS

150 GRAMS BEESWAX, GRATED

In a double boiler, simmer the herbs in the oil for twenty to forty minutes. Strain and return the oil to the pan, add the beeswax, and melt. Pour into warm glass jars. This is my preferred method.

You can also set an infused oil (see page 17) into a salve using this method. Slightly warm your prepared oil and add the beeswax, allowing two tablespoons of grated beeswax to 500 millilitres of infused oil after the herbal material has been strained off. Pour into shallow jars to set.

Coconut Balms

Coconut oil, solid at room temperature, is a perfect consistency for a simple balm. You can simply gently simmer your herbs at a low temperature in coconut oil for one to two hours, then strain into shallow jars to set. (I recently bought an electric chocolate melter from a discount supermarket for a few pounds, and this is perfect for the job.) Coconut adds its own benefits to a balm: it is anti-inflammatory and can reduce pain and swelling. It is intensely moisturising and contains antimicrobial lipids, lauric acid, capric acid, and caprylic acid, which have antifungal, antibacterial, and antiviral properties.

Compresses and Poultices

Compresses and poultices are a way of applying the benefits of herbs externally to the skin.

For a compress, soak a clean cotton cloth in a strong hot herbal infusion or decoction. Use this as hot as possible on the affected area (take care and do not burn yourself). Cover with a warm towel and leave for thirty minutes, and change the compress as it cools down by resoaking it in the infusion. Use one to two times a day.

Whereas a compress uses a cloth soaked in a liquid herbal infusion, a poultice employs herbs directly applied to the skin and then covered with a warm cloth. Use a mortar and pestle to bruise fresh herbs, apply directly to the skin, and cover with a warm cloth. Use one to two times a day.

Infused Oils

Fats and oils extract the oily and resinous properties of a herb, and these are often the antibacterial, antifungal, and wound-healing components. Infused oils are used for external applications. Unlike essential oils, they do not need to be diluted for use.

COLD INFUSED OIL (FOLK METHOD)

To make a cold infused oil, cut up the herb, place in a glass bottle or jar, and cover with vegetable oil such as olive, sunflower, almond, etc. Leave on a sunny windowsill for two weeks, shaking daily. Strain into a clean jar. This will keep in a cool, dark place for up to a year.

HEAT-MACERATED OIL (FOLK METHOD)

A hot maceration is quicker to make than a cold oil infusion. In a double boiler, put in the chopped herb and cover with a vegetable oil. Simmer very gently, covered, for two hours. Turn off the heat and allow the oil to cool before straining. If you wish, you can add fresh herbs to the oil and repeat the process for a stronger oil.

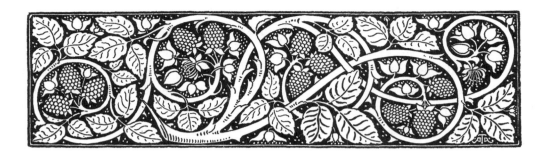

Cosmetic Uses of Herbs

It is reasonably easy and very satisfying to make your own organic, chemical-free, and eco-friendly personal care and beauty products. For the purposes of natural cosmetics and toiletries, fresh plants have more concentrated properties than dried ones, but both can be used. As well as herbs and spices, you can include other kitchen ingredients such as olive oil, honey, milk, cider vinegar, and so on.

Safety First

Even with the most pure and natural ingredients, it is still possible that some people will have an allergic or sensitive reaction. When using any new product or ingredient, it is advisable to carry out a patch test by placing a tiny amount of the product on the inside of your arm and monitoring it for any adverse reactions such as itching, reddening, soreness, or a rash. If this occurs, discontinue using the product.

Herbal Hair Rinses

Just as herbs can be beneficial for your health, they can have great benefits for your hair too. Choose the right ones and they can nourish the hair and scalp, boost circulation in your scalp, treat dandruff, cleanse, smooth the hair shaft, add shine, moisturise, reduce excess oil, restore the pH balance, remove odours, and promote hair growth. Some herbs will even bring out natural colours and highlights.

Hair rinses are really easy to make and use. If you can make a cup of tea, you can make a hair rinse. Simply bring 250 millilitres of water to boil in a saucepan, add a tablespoon of herbs, and turn off the heat. Allow this to cool down to room temperature and infuse overnight or for several hours at least. Strain, discarding the herbs and retaining the liquid. Once you have prepared your herbal hair rinse, it will keep in the fridge for three or four days.

To use, wash your hair as usual and rinse well with warm water. Have your hair rinse ready in a jug or, better still, a spray bottle. Spritz it on your hair and massage it gently through your hair and into your scalp. Leave it on for at least five minutes.

If you have only used herbs, you don't need to rinse this out and can go on to style your hair as usual. If you have added cider vinegar or lemon juice, you will need to rinse again with warm water.

As well as your herbs and spices, try adding cider vinegar, which is marvellous for removing product buildup from hair. Just add a couple tablespoons of cider vinegar to a pint of water and use this as a rinse, or add a tablespoon of cider vinegar to your prepared herbal hair rinse. It's great for removing excess oil from greasy hair, too, and will leave it shiny, soft, and silky. Also, you can add a tablespoon of lemon juice to a cup of water or add it to your prepared herbal hair rinse to treat greasy hair and stimulate hair growth. Over time, this will lighten your hair colour.

Facial Scrubs

Exfoliating is one of the most important things you can do to improve the condition of your skin. It gets rid of the old, dead cells that clog and dull it, rejuvenating your skin and leaving it glowing. Afterwards, your moisturiser and skin treatments will be better absorbed. Ground spices, herbs, almonds, fine oatmeal and bran, and even fresh ground coffee (the tannin reduces puffiness) can be effectively used as a gentle alternative to commercial chemical products, but please do not use salt on your face, though it is fine for a body scrub. You can experiment by adding carrier oils, eggs, honey, and tiny amounts of essential oils for extra benefits. Always avoid the delicate eye area when using a facial scrub.

Facial Steams

Facial steams help to deep cleanse your skin by opening the pores so that impurities are removed. It is especially useful if you have dull skin, blemishes or clogged pores, and even more effective if you follow the steam immediately with a face mask, then tone and moisturise. You can use hot water alone, but for added benefits you can add herbs. Start with a clean face. Put a heatproof bowl on a mat and fill it with boiling water, add your chosen herbs, leave them to infuse for a few minutes, and then put a towel over your head and lean over the bowl to let the steam work on your face for about ten minutes, taking a break when you need to. You can then follow with a mask or just wash your face with cool water to close the pores.

Face Masks

Face masks have a deep cleansing effect that removes toxins, impurities, and dead skin cells, as well as unclogs your pores. They help to improve skin tone and are an important part of any anti-aging or blemish-busting regime. Afterwards, your moisturiser will be better absorbed too. Herbal face masks employ herbs mixed with other ingredients, such as honey or yoghurt (soy or coconut yoghurt is fine), to help them "stick" to the skin. Alternatively, you can add some herbal infusion to cosmetic clay (available on the internet). Face masks, especially natural ones, can be very, very messy, so it's a good idea to apply them while you are in the bath. Cleanse your face first; if possible, use a herbal steam to open your pores. Apply the mask to the damp skin of your neck and face, avoiding the delicate eye area. Relax while the mask sets, leave it for the recommended time, and then wash the mask away with plenty of warm water and a washcloth. Follow with your favourite moisturiser.

Skin Toners

Using a toner after cleansing helps to remove any oily residue left by your cleanser as well as tone and refine the skin. You can combine herb and spice infusions and decoctions with witch hazel, rose water, or cider vinegar.

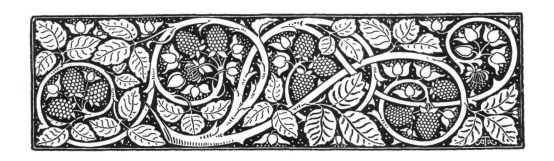

Your Magical Workshop

R un out of some magical ingredient and need to work a spell or ritual in a hurry? You can use your kitchen herbs and spices in your magical and spiritual work.

Equipment Needed

- Pestle and mortar
- Bottles and jars
- Kitchen scales
- Measuring jug
- Ribbons, string, wire
- Cloth or bags
- Candles
- Charcoal blocks

The Magical Virtues of Plants

Each ingredient possesses its own virtues and energies. It has its own vibration, depending on its characteristics, makeup, and the environment it grew in, taking in nutrients from its surroundings and energy from the sun, becoming a unique being. Always remember that you are working with the virtues inherent in the plant to achieve the result you want, whether that is to evoke the energy of a particular deity or season or for protection, cleansing, love, purification, abundance, and so on. These are known as a plant's correspondences, and at the heading of each herb in the A–Z herbal are the correspondences for the planetary ruler, element, and associated deities, followed by the plant's magical virtues.

Let's look briefly at what some of those things mean.

THE PLANETS

SUN: The sun is dynamic and expansive. Herbs ruled by the sun turn towards the sun or have yellow flowers. The sun rules over prosperity and general protection.

MARS: Mars is the planet of war, so Mars plants symbolise a warlike spirit and generally have thorns or stings. Mars energy is assertive, spontaneous, and daring.

SATURN: Saturn is the planet of aging, limitation, and death, so Saturn plants are slow growing or long living and woody, thrive in the shade and have deep roots, or are poisonous, foul smelling, or considered evil. Saturn's energy is to do with limitation, change, the crystallisation of efforts, and endings. Because this is a kitchen herbal, very few of the plants in this book fall under Saturn.

MERCURY: Mercury is the planet of communication, so Mercury plants include fast-growing weeds, creepers and winding plants, or plants with hairy, fuzzy, or finely divided leaves. They may be aromatic. Mercury energy rules the mind and intellect.

VENUS: Venus is the planet of love and beauty, so Venus plants overwhelm the senses with sweet scents and lovely flowers, red fruits, or soft, furry leaves. Venus energy is feminine, creative, harmonious, and loving.

MOON: The moon governs the tides, and moon plants often grow near water or have a high water content or juicy leaves. They may have white flowers or moon-shaped leaves or seed pods. Moon energy is subtle, feminine, and inward looking. The moon rules the instinct, emotions, and psychic abilities.

JUPITER: Jupiter is the bringer of abundance, so Jupiter plants are usually big and bold and often edible. Jupiter is benign, expansive, and optimistic.

THE ELEMENTS

EARTH: The powers of earth are concerned with what is manifest: the material, the fixed, the solid, and the practical; with what is rooted. Earth magic is concerned with manifestation, business, health, practicality, wealth, stability, grounding and centring, fertility and agriculture. Earth plants tend to be nourishing or earthy smelling.

AIR: The powers of air are concerned with the intellect, the powers of the mind, knowledge (as opposed to wisdom), logic, inspiration, information, teaching, memory, thought, and communication. Air magic is usually concerned with the intellectual or the spiritual, and in ritual air is symbolised through the use of perfume or incense. Air plants are often freshly fragrant, such as mint.

WATER: Water is associated with the emotions, feelings, and the subconscious, and water magic is usually concerned with divination and scrying. Water plants are juicy and fleshy or grow near water.

FIRE: Fire magic is concerned with creativity, life energy, and zeal. Fire gives us vitality, igniting action, animation, and movement. It sparks courage and acts of bravery. It heats passion and enthusiasm. Fire is the power of inner sight and creative vision, directing it and controlling it to make it manifest in the world. Fire plants tend to have fiery sap or a hot taste, like ginger, or warm perfumes, such as clove and cinnamon.

DEITY CORRESPONDENCES

Various religions have assigned specific plants to different gods and used them in the worship of those deities or associated them in mythology. Where I have assigned gods and goddesses to herbs, it is because those plants were connected with those particular deities either in their mythology or worship. They are not arbitrarily assigned.

Incorporating Herbs in Magic

There are numerous ways you can incorporate the energy of a herb into your spiritual and magical practice, and here are just a few:

LIVING ENERGY PRESENCE

Simply having a herb growing on your kitchen windowsill will bring the living energy of that plant into your home. Some plants, such as basil, are believed to be protective spirits in their own right.

DISPLAYED FOR MAGICAL PURPOSES

The energy of a herb can be brought into your environment by creating a herbal talisman or herbal charm bag, always concentrating on your purpose and intent and then hanging it in the place it is most needed, such as the kitchen or bedroom. Hang a string of dried chillies or garlic in your kitchen as a protective charm, sprigs of dill for peace, a lemon pomander to dispel evil, and so on.

WREATHS

A wreath is simply an arrangement of flowers or leaves woven into a ring. To make one, you can use a wire, wicker, or foam circle (these are available from florists or online) as a base, or just twist woodier herbs together and secure with wire or ribbon. Hang a wreath on your front door to protect the magical threshold between inside and outside and prevent negativity from entering. Depending on what herbs and flowers you use, wreaths can also be worn during rituals, celebrations, and feasts, hung above the bed, or laid on graves.

CARRY ABOUT THE PERSON

Throughout the ages, people have put leaves of particular herbs in their pockets or purses when they wanted to carry the energy of that herb with them. Carry "lucky basil" to attract abundance, rosemary to deflect ill will, sage for protection, and so on.

PLACED UNDER THE PILLOW

Placing a herb beneath the pillow to absorb its energy is an ancient practice. Coriander was placed beneath the pillow as an aphrodisiac, garlic for protection, rosemary for prophetic dreams, and so on.

CHARM BAGS

This is one of the simplest forms of magic using herbs. Herbal charm bags are fabric pouches filled with dried herbs. You can either buy a pouch (wedding favour bags work well) or, better still, make one yourself. It doesn't have to be a work of art; it is the intent that is important. You will need an oblong piece of cloth, big enough to take all the ingredients when folded in half and sewn up. Choose a sturdy fabric, and the right colour adds extra strength to the magic (see appendix 2). Take the cloth and fold it in half, right sides together. Sew up three sides, reinforcing your intent with each stitch (you can chant it as you sew), and then turn it right-side out. Put the ingredients into the pouch one by one, stating your desire each time. You can blend several different dried herbs to suit your purpose. Sew it shut, and then either carry it with you, put it in the appropriate room of your house, or sleep with it under your pillow, according to its purpose.

ASPERGERS (SPRINKLERS)

Aspergers are sprinklers made from woody herb stems such as sage, rosemary, or mint used for scattering consecrated water or herbal infusions in order to purify a place or person of negative vibrations and energies. To make one, take some fresh sprigs of herbs about 15 centimetres (6 inches) long and bind them together at one end using white thread. To use the asperger, dip it into the liquid and sprinkle it around the area (a circle, temple, house, or shop, for example) or person to be purified.

POTIONS

Potion is a generic term for herbal preparations made in a ritual way. They are made according to the same methods as infusions and decoctions made for healing, but brewed with magical intent, preferably at the correct moon phase and season and perhaps with appropriate words and symbolic actions.

The simplest way to brew a herbal potion is akin to making a cup of tea. Take your herb, put it in a pot, and pour on boiling water. Hold the vessel in your hands and imbue it with your intent. Strain and use. Some potions are used on external objects, while some are drunk. The purpose of a potion depends on the herbs chosen. You can use consecration herbs to consecrate magical objects, a purification potion can be used with an asperger to purify the temple or working area, a banishing potion can be used to cleanse a place of negative energies, and so on.

EATEN OR DRUNK

When you ingest a herb, you make an intimate connection with it, absorbing its vibrational energy into your body and your own energy field, changing its frequency; it becomes part of you forever. When you do this with intent, consciously, as part of spiritual practice or ritual, it becomes a communion of spirits. Herbs can be consumed in teas, potions, food, or infused in wine.

PHILTRES

Philtre is the specific name for a love potion, used to make one person fall in love with another. Modern witches believe it to be very wrong to manipulate the will of another. Instead, it is permissible to ask for love to come to you and let the universe decide who it shall be. A philtre can be a simple one-herb tea or a blend of several herbs of love or a wine or mead made or infused with appropriate herbs.

THE RITUAL CUP

The dedication of the bread and wine is one of the central points of every Pagan ritual. Wine is one of the "god containing" substances believed by the ancients to allow people to share in God consciousness. The cup that contains the wine symbolises the cauldron or grail, which contains wisdom and inspiration. The chalice of wine and the platter of bread are passed around the circle with the words "blessed be" to be shared by all present with love and blessings. This intimate act creates a connection with every other person present as well as a communion with the gods. Herbs infused in wine, or wine made with herbs, can be used as a ritual drink. You will need to tailor the herbs used to your purpose for different sabbats and events such as handfastings.

POWDERS

Herbs, barks, and roots can be powdered together for use in magic. You can scatter a powder around your house or possessions to protect them, put a pinch of money-drawing powder in your purse, put them in charm bags, sprinkle them on candles, or use them to consecrate tools and amulets.

HELD IN RITUAL

When working ritual, you can call on the appropriate herbal energies by wearing a wreath of herbs or carrying a sprig of herbs into the circle.

OFFERINGS

When performing spells and rituals, it is customary to make offerings to the gods and spirits. Such offerings can take the form of bread and cakes baked with suitable herbs left in the ritual venue, incense, libations of herbal wines, or simply bunches of herbs left in the places you work to thank the spirits for their help. Please never leave wire, ribbons, or plastic tied to these as this is just littering and the spirits will not be pleased.

IN CONJUNCTION WITH CANDLES

Infused oils can be used to anoint the candles used in candle magic, or you can stud a candle with spices such as cloves (do be careful because as they burn they can explode), or warm the outside of the candle and then roll it in dried herbs. This adds the energy of the herbs to a ritual or spell, or you can perform a candle magic spell. For this, decide what spell you wish to work and choose a candle in the appropriate colour. Set it up on a low table one evening and put out most of the lights in the room. Take the corresponding herb-infused oil and anoint the candle middle to top and middle to bottom with the oil, concentrating on what you want to achieve. When you are satisfied, light the candle and state your purpose. Leave it to burn itself out (make sure it is in a safe place).

INCENSE

Everyone knows that witches and magicians use incenses during rituals—powerful perfumes that help the magic. They may be stimulating or calming, soothing or invigorating, raise or depress the spirits. You can use your kitchen herbs and spices in your ritual incenses. Loose incense is probably the easiest type of incense to make and the most useful kind for magical ritual. All the measurements in this book are by volume, not weight, and I use a spoon to measure out small quantities when I am making a single jar of incense or a cup for large quantities and big batches. Therefore, if the recipe says three parts rosemary, a half part thyme, and one part oregano, this means three spoons of rosemary, half a spoon of thyme, and one spoon of oregano. If using resins and essential oils, these should be combined together first, stirring lightly with the pestle and left to go a little sticky before you add any woods, barks, and crushed berries. Next add any herbs and powders and lastly any flowers.

To use your incenses, take a self-igniting charcoal block (available from occult and church suppliers) and apply a match to it. It will begin to spark across its surface and eventually glow red. Place it on a flame-proof dish with a mat underneath (it will get very hot). When the charcoal block is glowing, sprinkle a pinch of the incense on top; a little goes a long way. Alternatively, if you are celebrating outdoors and have a bonfire, you can throw much larger quantities of incense directly onto the flames.

For incense to be burned indoors, I generally add resins like frankincense or myrrh to improve the scent and burning quality, but if I am working outdoors I will just use a blend of herbs that I throw on the bonfire.

SMUDGE

If you feel that your home has accumulated negative energy or if there is a bad atmosphere lingering after an argument, you can take several measures to cleanse it. (It is a good idea to do this on a regular basis in any case.) One of the simplest ways of cleansing your home of negative energy is to use a smudge stick as you walk from room to room. Smudging also can be used to cleanse the aura and any magical tools or ritual objects.

RITUAL OILS

Infused oils made from herbs and spices can be used in spells and rituals to anoint people and candles and to consecrate tools, talismans, amulets, and so on.

FLOWER ESSENCES

A flower essence is the bioenergetic imprint of a flower transmitted by a process of solarisation to water, which then holds the memory of the plant's vibrational essence. Flower essences work on energy pathways to heal on an emotional, mental, and spiritual level, and the spiritual aspect of the remedies is why I have included flower essences in this section. They were pioneered by Edward Bach, an English surgeon who believed that disease was the end result of internal emotional, mental, and spiritual conflict, and therefore the cure for any illness also needed to address these. He created thirty-eight flower remedies (though many more have been researched since), using them as gentle, natural vibrational catalysts to return the spirit to harmony.

Flower essences are simple to prepare and very safe to use. Gather a few mature flowers. Float them on the surface of 150 millilitres spring water in a bowl and leave in the sun for three to four hours. Make sure that they are not shadowed in any way. Remove the flowers. Pour the water into a bottle and top up with 150 millilitres brandy or vodka to preserve it. This is your mother essence. To make up your flower essences for use, put seven drops from this into a 10-millilitre dropper bottle, and top that up with brandy or vodka. This is your dosage bottle. The usual dose is four drops of this in a glass of water four times a day. When making flower essences, it is important not to handle the flowers. You want the vibrational imprint of the flowers to be held by the water, not your own imprint.

IN CONJUNCTION WITH MEDITATION

The vibrational energy of herbs can be helpful in your meditation practice and chakra work. Try holding a sprig or leaf of a particular herb within your aura as you meditate.

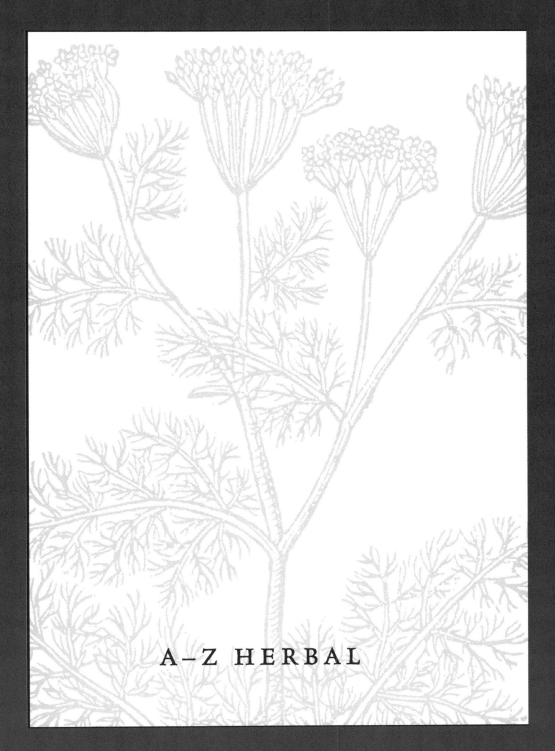

A–Z HERBAL

Basil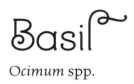

Ocimum spp.

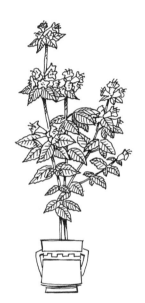

PLANETARY RULER: Mars

ELEMENT: Fire

ASSOCIATED DEITIES: Erzulie, Aphrodite, Krishna, Lakshmi, Vishnu, Jesus, Virgin Mary, Saint Joseph, Dhanvantari

MAGICAL VIRTUES: Blessing, peace, harmony, protection, resurrection, dispelling negativity, exorcism, healing, love, luck, wealth

In Hinduism, the holy basil—called *tulsi* or *tulasi*—is regarded the holiest of all plants, the threshold between heaven and earth.[3] There are many stories as to how tulsi came into being, and in all of them the plant has a divine origin. In one Hindu legend, Dhanvantari, the physician of the gods, shed tears of joy that transformed into the tulsi plant.[4] Tulsi is most often regarded as a manifestation of Lakshmi, the goddess of wealth, and in Hindu homes tulsi is revered as a household deity; there is a common belief that where Tulasi Devi ("the goddess Tulasi") resides, auspicious vibrations, peace, and prosperity always dwell.[5] All forms of ghosts and demons run away from the place where Tulasi Devi is planted, and all kinds of sinful reactions are destroyed when one comes close to Tulasi

3   Simoons, *Plants of Life, Plants of Death.*
4   Aruna Deshpande, *India: A Divine Destination* (Crest Publishing House, 2005).
5   Swami Vibhooti Saraswati, *Tulasi—India's Most Sacred Plant*, http://www.yogamag.net/archives/2006
      /koct06/tulsi.shtml, accessed 11 April 17.

Devi.[6] Growing a basil plant brings a sacred energy to your home; in Hinduism, holy basil is considered to be the Mother Goddess incarnated in plant form, a protective spirit that deflects negative energy from its surroundings, bringing peace, prosperity, and blessings.

The Greek Orthodox Church also considers basil to be the holiest herb of all. It is said that when Helena, mother of the Roman emperor Constantine the Great, was seeking the True Cross at Golgotha in 326 CE, she noticed a patch of basil growing in the corner of a disused temple of Aphrodite.[7] As basil means "of the king" in Greek, and she was looking for traces of Christ, who is called the "king of kings" by Christians, she saw this as a sign and ordered the excavations begun on the spot. The diggers found a piece of wood with a sprig of basil growing from it. To test this, Helena asked some sick people to touch it, and when they were healed, she knew this was a fragment of the True Cross.[8]

On January 6 the faithful of the Orthodox Church attend the Great Feast of the Theophany, when the congregation receives holy water in small bottles. Later, they invite the priest to bless their homes with this holy water by dipping a sprig of basil into it and sprinkling it about the house. This is believed to be so powerful that it will rid the house of evil spirits and even the Kallikantzaroi, the malign spirits of chaos who appear during the Twelve Days of Christmas,[9] are driven away on the Eve of the Epiphany by a priest with holy water and a basil sprinkler.[10]

A basil plant helps remove negative energies from the home, its pure energy cleanses the space. It is used for warding off harmful spiritual energies, evil spirits, black magic, and psychic attacks. Grow one by the front door to prevent unwanted influences coming in, or keep one in the kitchen to foster domestic harmony. To cleanse your house or sacred space, make **Basil Tea** and sprinkle it with a fresh sprig of basil in all the corners of each room. This may be useful when you move into a new house and are aware of unwanted vibrations left by the previous tenants.

Basil is also useful for dispelling mental and spiritual negativity. Take a cup of **Basil Tea** each day for seven days or use **Basil Flower Essence** for twenty-one days. You can also add a couple drops of **Basil Flower Essence** to your bath. Protect yourself when you know you are going to be facing a difficult situation by dabbing a spot of **Basil Infused Oil** onto your forehead.

---

6   http://www.gutenberg.org/files/44638/44638-h/44638-h.htm#chapter-5, accessed 11 April 17.
7   https://orthodoxwiki.org/Elevation_of_the_Holy_Cross, accessed 11 April 17.
8   Brannon Parker, *The Serpent, the Eagle, the Lion and the Disk* (Lulu.com, 2012).
9   Anna Franklin, *Yule, History, Lore and Celebration* (Lear Books, 2010).
10   Simoons, *Plants of Life, Plants of Death.*

In Europe basil seems to have had a mixed reputation. Nicolas Culpeper[11] recommended that it should be applied to the stings of venomous beasts to draw out the poison, on the principle that "like draws like," as he thought of basil as a malign herb and assigned it to the planet Mars and the sign of Scorpio the scorpion. This may have been because in hot countries it was observed that scorpions liked to shelter beneath pots of basil, and this gave rise to the superstition that a sprig of basil left beneath a pot would turn into a scorpion or that bruised basil plants would yield scorpions. Despite what Culpeper wrote, in Tudor England basil was considered a lucky and protective plant, and it was often a gift to a couple setting up house or given as a parting gift to guests.[12] Follow this tradition by presenting a pot of basil to friends setting up home, along with a blessing.

Basil is widely associated with love and sexual arousal. In Ayurveda basil is considered an aphrodisiac, while the Roman author Pliny recommended its use at the time of mating horses and donkeys. In Tuscany basil is called *amorino*, or "little love," while in central Italy it is called *Bacia-nicola* ("kiss me Nicholas"). In some districts of Italy, girls wore basil behind their ears when visiting their sweethearts.[13] Basil resonates with the energy of love. Use in love spells, love incense, and charm bags. Wear **Basil Infused Oil** to attract a lover.

Basil is one of the few herbs that can be used to help balance all of the chakras, as well as purify the aura and align the body's energy field. Use **Basil Infused Oil** to anoint the chakras in daily practice, and spend a few minutes meditating with a basil leaf held between your palms at the level of the heart chakra to open your heart to love and compassion.

The belief in basil as a wealth-attracting herb is also widespread. In India it represents Lakshmi, the goddess of wealth. In the West Indies basil is sprinkled around new business premises to ensure good fortune for the enterprise. Some Mexicans still carry "lucky basil" in a pocket or purse to magnetize money. Basil resonates with the flow of abundance. Carry a basil leaf in your purse, eat a basil leaf, or dab some **Basil Infused Oil** on your forehead before you go out to find new work or start a new venture. If you have a business, place a basil leaf in the cash register to attract plenty, and sprinkle **Basil Tea** or some dried, powdered basil herb over the threshold of your premises to attract customers.

---

11 *Culpeper's Complete Herbal.*
12 http://www.gardenersworld.com/plants/plant-inspiration/fact-file-basil, accessed 11 April 17.
13 Angelo de Gubernatis, *La Mythologie Des Plantes: Ou, Les Legendes Du Regne Vegetal* (Scholar's Choice edition, 2015).

CULINARY USES

Often known as "the king of the culinary herbs," basil has been used for cooking since ancient times and was a staple herb in the kitchen gardens of ancient Greece and Rome.[14] Basil is used in stews, salads, soups, sauces, vegetable dishes, and pesto. There are more than 150 varieties of this extraordinary plant, but most culinary basils are cultivars of sweet basil (*Ocinum basilicum*), including Genovese basil (*O. basilicum* 'Genovese"), Thai basil (*O. basilicum* var. *thyrsiflora*), and cinnamon basil (*O. basilicum* 'Cinnamon"). Other species include holy basil, also called tulsi or tulasi (*O. sanctum* syn. *O. tenuiflorum*) and lemon basil (*O. americanum*). If you are cooking with basil, it is always best to use it fresh and add it towards the end of the cooking process to retain the scent and flavour of its volatile oils.

COSMETIC USES

Basil contain antioxidants that help protect your skin from the oxidative stress and the free radical damage that leads to fine lines and wrinkles. It also helps tighten the skin, improve its tone, and boost the growth of new skin cells. To get the benefits of basil, you can simply massage **Basil Tea** into your skin and rinse off with warm water once a day. Use **Basil Infused Oil** as a moisturising treatment. Once a week, make a basil face pack by blitzing a handful of fresh basil leaves into a paste and applying directly to your face and neck, mixed with honey or yoghurt if desired. Leave for fifteen to twenty minutes and wash off with lukewarm water. Follow with a moisturiser.

MEDICINAL USES

ACTIONS: Anthelminthic, anticatarrhal, antidysmenorrhea, antifungal, anti-inflammatory, antimicrobial, antioxidant, antispasmodic, antiviral, carminative, demulcent, digestive, expectorant, hypotensive, insecticidal

Basil has been used in traditional and folk medicine for thousands of years. In Ayurvedic medicine, tulsi (holy basil) is considered to be the most powerful of all medicinal plants, and Hindu mythology says that even Yama, the god of death, gives way to holy tulsi. Despite the glut of articles appearing about the almost miraculous healing powers of tulsi, holy basil and sweet basil actually have very similar medicinal qualities.

The pungent scent and strong flavour of basil tell us that it is packed full of volatile oils. These vary in quantity and proportion depending on the cultivar; sweet basil has a strong clove scent because of its high concentration of eugenol, for example, while lemon basil

---

14   Pliny the Elder, *The Natural History*.

has a strong citrus scent owing to its concentration of limonene. Currently, there are many studies looking into the medicinal properties of basil and basil essential oil, and these are very promising. In the lab, basil has been shown to have antimicrobial, antiviral, antifungal, insecticidal, antioxidant, anti-aging and anti-inflammatory activity.[15] So adding some basil to your diet can't hurt but may reap many health benefits!

There are several herbs with anti-inflammatory properties that can help arthritis, some of which have been shown to be as effective as non-steroidal anti-inflammatory drugs (NSAIDs), and basil is one of these.[16] Drink a cup or two of **Basil Tea** daily, and externally use a **Basil Hot Compress** or warmed **Basil Infused Oil** on affected areas.

Basil contains anti-itching compounds such as thymol and camphene (the latter also has a cooling effect) that can help eczema. Using basil with a vegetable oil will help keep the skin moisturised and supple, which is also important when treating this condition, so smooth on **Basil Infused Oil** or apply a paste of pulverised fresh basil leaves mixed with an equal quantity of vegetable oil.

Basil is considered to be a mild antidepressant as well as an adaptogen, a herbal medicine that helps the body normalize the harmful effects of stressors.[17] Make a cup of **Basil Tea** and sip it during the day when you are feeling stress, or pour a cup of **Basil Infusion** into a soothing bath to unwind after a difficult day.

Basil has a mildly sedative action. Drink a cup of **Basil Tea** before bed to help get you off to sleep.

Studies have shown that basil has antibacterial properties, and a wash of **Basil Infusion** can be employed externally for ulcers, cuts, and wounds. The antifungal properties make it a useful mouthwash and gargle for oral thrush.

---

15   H. R. Juliani and J. E. Simon, "Antioxidant Activity of Basil" in J. Janick and A. Whipkey (eds.), *Trends in New Crops and New Uses* (Alexandria, VA: ASHS Press), 575–579, https://hort.purdue.edu/newcrop /ncnu02/v5-575.html, accessed 29 February 17.

16   Jürg Gertsch, Marco Leonti, Stefan Raduner, Ildiko Racz, Jian-Zhong Chen, Xiang-Qun Xie, Karl-Heinz Altmann, Meliha Karsak, and Andreas Zimmer, "Beta-caryophyllene Is a Dietary Cannabinoid," *Proceedings of the National Academy of Sciences* 105, no. 26 (July 2008): 9099–9104, DOI: 10.1073 /pnas.0803601105. A. Vijayalaxmi, Vasudha Bakshi, and Nazia Begum, "Anti-Arthritic and Anti-Inflammatory Activity of Beta Caryophyllene Against Freund's Complete Adjuvant Induced Arthritis in Wistar Rats," *Journal of Bone Reports and Recommendations*, http://bone.imedpub.com/antiarthritic -and-anti-inflammatory-activity-of-beta-caryophyllene-against-freunds-complete-adjuvant-induced -arthritis-in-wistar-rats.php?aid=7220, accessed 29 March 17.

17   S. Joti, S. Satendra, S. Sushma, T. Anjana, and S. Shashi, "Antistressor Activity of *Ocimum sanctum* (Tulsi) Against Experimentally Induced Oxidative Stress in Rabbits," https://www.ncbi.nlm.nih.gov /pubmed/17922070, DOI: 10.1358/mf.2007.29.6.1118135, accessed 7 April 17.

CAUTION: Basil is generally recognised as safe in food amounts and likely safe in medicinal amounts for most people, but do not take medicinal amounts of basil for more than four weeks. However, basil lowers blood sugar and blood pressure marginally, so use medicinal amounts with care if you are on medications for diabetes or hypertension. It may slow blood clotting, so avoid medicinal amounts for at least two weeks before surgery or if you are already taking anticlotting medications. Medicinal amounts of basil should not be taken by pregnant or breastfeeding women. You may have read that a study conducted by the Bureau of Food and Drug Analysis discovered that safrole, a substance found in basil, induced liver cancer in rats when given in large quantities, but "you would have to eat kilograms of basil every day for years on end before having to start worrying about its carcinogenic properties," according to the researcher Wen Chi-Pang.[18]

18   http://www.taipeitimes.com/News/taiwan/archives/2007/05/15/2003360954, accessed 15 May 2017.

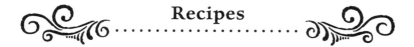

Recipes

BASIL TEA

250 MILLILITRES (1 CUP) BOILING WATER

4-5 FRESH BASIL LEAVES

Pour the boiling water over the leaves. Let it steep for four to five minutes. Strain and drink.

BASIL INFUSION

50 GRAMS (2 CUPS) CHOPPED FRESH BASIL

500 MILLILITRES (2 CUPS) BOILING WATER

Put the herbs in a pot and pour the boiling water on them. Cover and infuse for twenty minutes. Strain.

BASIL INFUSED OIL

Pack a sterilised glass jar with fresh, crushed basil leaves. Fill this up with vegetable oil, making sure the herb is covered. Fit the lid and leave on a sunny windowsill for two weeks, shaking daily. Strain the oil into a clean glass jar. Keep in a cool, dark place for up to a year.

BASIL HOT COMPRESS

Make a fresh **Basil Infusion**. While it is hot, dip in a clean cotton cloth and apply it as warm as you can bear to the affected part. When it cools, dip it in the infusion again and reapply. You can do this several times.

BASIL FLOWER ESSENCE

Gather six mature basil flowers. Float them on the surface of 150 millilitres spring water in a bowl and leave in the sun for three or four hours. Make sure that they are not shadowed in any way. Remove the flowers. Pour the water into a bottle and top up with 150 millilitres brandy or vodka to preserve it. This is your mother essence. To make up the flower essences for use, put seven drops from this into a 10-millilitre dropper bottle, and top that up with brandy or vodka. The usual dose is four drops of this in a glass of water four times a day.

BASIL VINEGAR

Put a few sprigs of fresh basil into a glass jar of cider vinegar. Fit a lid and leave on a sunny windowsill for two weeks, shaking daily. Strain the vinegar into a clean bottle. You can use this as a salad dressing, pour in your bath to cleanse you and help you relax, or use as a magical cleanser to clean tools, sacred spaces, and people.

BASIL SHAMPOO

250 MILLILITRES (1 CUP) BASIL INFUSION

150 MILLILITRES (10 TABLESPOONS) LIQUID CASTILE SOAP

3 MILLILITRES (½ TEASPOON) OLIVE OIL

8 DROPS BASIL ESSENTIAL OIL (OPTIONAL)

Combine the ingredients and bottle. Shake well before use. This will not lather as much as a commercial shampoo, but it will cleanse and treat your hair with nourishing basil. This will keep in the fridge for a week.

. . . .

BASIL SKIN TONER

25 BASIL LEAVES

200 MILLILITRES (¾ CUP) ROSE WATER

1 CENTIMETRE LEMON ZEST (NO WHITE PITH)

100 MILLILITRES (½ CUP) WITCH HAZEL

3 MILLILITRES (½ TEASPOON) BENZOIN TINCTURE

Put the basil, rose water, and lemon in a pan and warm gently for ten minutes. Do not boil. Remove from the heat and leave to infuse for three to four hours. Sieve through fine muslin into a jug or bowl and stir in the witch hazel and benzoin tincture (a preservative). Pour into a glass bottle, stopper, and store in the fridge for up to two weeks. Use morning and evening by dabbing it on your face and neck with a cotton wool pad. Follow with a moisturiser. This will help bust blemishes and deep clean, tighten, and protect your skin from environmental stresses. Basil is a powerful cleanser, and this toner is perfect for those with oily skin and clogged pores.

. . . .

BASIL AND EGG WHITE FACE MASK

8 BASIL LEAVES

WHITE OF 1 EGG, WHISKED

1 TEASPOON HONEY

Pulp the basil leaves finely in a blender or pestle and mortar. Add the juice to the whisked egg white and honey and apply to the skin of the face. Leave on for twenty to thirty minutes, then wash off with lukewarm water. Finish with a splash of cold water to close the pores, and apply your moisturiser. Basil and honey have antiseptic properties that help clear up the infections that cause blemishes, while the egg white helps to tighten the skin and reduce enlarged pores. Try adding one teaspoon of ground turmeric powder for an extra anti-inflammatory effect. This will also help remove blackheads.

. . . . .

Black Pepper

Piper nigrum

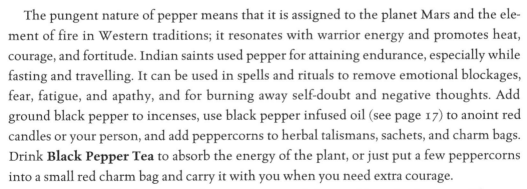

PLANETARY RULER: Mars

ELEMENT: Fire

ASSOCIATED DEITIES: Shakti, Lakshmi,[19]
Pana Narasimha,[20] Hanuman, Jagannath,
Subhadra, Balabhadra, Saint Anthony

MAGICAL VIRTUES: Banishing, protection, courage

The pungent nature of pepper means that it is assigned to the planet Mars and the element of fire in Western traditions; it resonates with warrior energy and promotes heat, courage, and fortitude. Indian saints used pepper for attaining endurance, especially while fasting and travelling. It can be used in spells and rituals to remove emotional blockages, fear, fatigue, and apathy, and for burning away self-doubt and negative thoughts. Add ground black pepper to incenses, use black pepper infused oil (see page 17) to anoint red candles or your person, and add peppercorns to herbal talismans, sachets, and charm bags. Drink **Black Pepper Tea** to absorb the energy of the plant, or just put a few peppercorns into a small red charm bag and carry it with you when you need extra courage.

The energy of black pepper relates to the root chakra and its primal energy. The root chakra connects us to the earth from which we receive all of the vital nutrients essential

---

19   Sharma, *Western Himalayan Temple Records.*
20   Knapp, *Krishna Deities and Their Miracles.*

to our survival; it grounds and stabilises us. Those people whose root chakras are closed or underactive tend to be fearful, nervous, anxious, disconnected, or depressed. Those whose root chakras are overactive tend to be aggressive and materialistic. However, the root chakra is the foundation from which all is built, where the goddess Shakti, in the form of kundalini energy, lies coiled. Help balance the root chakra by including black pepper in your diet, anointing the chakra with black pepper infused oil (see page 17), or while meditating on your connection to Mother Earth and your trust in her to nurture you.

In Hindi black pepper is known as *marich*, one of the names for the sun, as it is thought to be filled with solar energy. At the Makar Sankranti festival, which marks the end of the winter solstice month in January and reverences the sun god Surya,[21] people prepare special sweet rice made with sugar, banana, coconut, and black pepper. It is used as an offering to Hindu gods such as Lakshmi,[22] Pana Narasimha,[23] Hanuman, Jagannath, Subhadra, and Balabhadra. Black pepper is also known as *kali mirri* (literally "black pepper" and not to be confused with the goddess Kali).

In some traditions, black pepper is used to combat spirit possession. Islamic exorcists use ingredients like lime, vinegar, black pepper, and ginger, which are thought to burn *jinn* (spirits), in conjunction with prayers to drive jinni from a victim's body.[24] You can add black pepper to incense used for exorcism and banishing or combine with salt and sprinkle it around boundaries to prevent psychic attack and dispel negative influences. Combine with dried sage and burn as incense to remove bad energies from a new home or office.

CULINARY USES

Just as basil is called "king of herbs," black pepper is called "king of spices." It is hard to imagine now, but it was once one of the most valuable commodities in the world, worth its weight in gold. When Alaric the Visigoth besieged Rome in 408 CE, he demanded 2,500 kilograms of pepper as part of the ransom.[25] In the Middle Ages, land tenants even paid their rent in pepper.[26] This led to the symbolic handing over of a peppercorn to confirm a

---

21   J. Gordon Melton, *Religious Celebrations: An Encyclopedia of Holidays, Festivals, Solemn Observances, and Spiritual Commemorations*, 2011.

22   Sharma, *Western Himalayan Temple Records*.

23   Knapp, *Krishna Deities and Their Miracles*.

24   http://islamicexorcism.com, accessed 17 October 17.

25   Swain, *The Lore of Spices*.

26   Ibid.

relationship of tenancy, which led to the expression "peppercorn rent," but as peppercorns fell in value, this came to mean an insignificant fee.[27]

The word *pepper* comes from the Sanskrit *pippali,* meaning "berry."[28] Black, white, and green peppercorns all come from the same plant, but they are harvested at different stages of maturity. Green peppercorns are picked while the berries are still unripe and green. Black peppercorns are harvested as the fruit starts to turn red and left to sun dry, shrivel, and turn black, while white peppercorns are ripe berries soaked in brine, which removes the outer skin to expose the white-coloured seed.

Black pepper is one of the most versatile cooking spices, used in soups, stews, marinades and pickles. Its pungent flavour comes from its volatile oils, but these are lost when the pepper is milled and stored, so it is always best to grind pepper just before use.

COSMETIC USES

Crush black peppercorns and use to make a **Black Pepper Exfoliating Facial Scrub** that will remove dead cells from the skin and bring blood to the surface, leaving your skin healthy and glowing. This will help it absorb more nutrients from your moisturiser. The antibacterial and anti-inflammatory qualities of black pepper are especially helpful if you suffer from acne.

MEDICINAL USES

ACTIONS: carminative, decongestant, expectorant, anti-inflammatory

Traditional Indian Ayurvedic medicine uses tiny amounts of black pepper to make the other herbs in the formula more available to the body. We now know that one of the most important benefits of black pepper is that it enhances the bioavailability of phytochemicals from other spices and herbs, such as turmeric, as well as vitamins and minerals.[29]

In Ayurvedic medicine black pepper is believed to kindle *agni,* the digestive fire. Like many aromatic kitchen herbs, black pepper is considered a carminative in Western herbalism; in other words, it stimulates digestion and intestinal motility to ease gas and bloating. The taste of black pepper on the tongue triggers the stomach to release hydrochloric acid, needed for the digestive process. If the body fails to produce enough, an inefficient

---

27 Ibid.
28 Sesha T. R. Iyengar, *Dravidian India* (Asian Educational Services, 2000).
29 G. B. Dudhatra et al., "A Comprehensive Review on Pharmacotherapeutics of Herbal Bioenhancers," *The Scientific World Journal,* 2012.

digestive process may lead to heartburn or indigestion, so adding a little black pepper to food may help alleviate these problems.

Black pepper is a warming spice, its pungency due to one of its active compounds, piperine, which increases the production of heat in the body.[30] Black pepper boosts the metabolism, and a little black pepper can help in the fight against obesity.

Black pepper is a natural painkiller. It sounds counterintuitive, but sprinkling black pepper powder onto a cut will slow down bleeding and have painkilling, antiseptic, and antibiotic properties. Black pepper can be applied directly to the skin in the form of a **Black Pepper Compress** for treating nerve pain (neuralgia). It has long been used as a home remedy for toothache by applying a little freshly ground black pepper to the tooth and gums. Black pepper is an excellent anti-inflammatory agent; piperine reduces the inflammatory compounds that make arthritic pain worse, so try adding a little black pepper to your food, and use a **Black Pepper Compress** on affected parts.

Black pepper is a decongestant, useful in the treatment of colds, coughs, and flu, as well as being an expectorant, which means it helps break up congestion in the chest and sinuses. Fight off the seasonal misery with **Black Pepper Tea** or try taking a teaspoon of antiseptic **Fire Cider** every day in the winter as a preventative.

CAUTION: Black pepper is considered to be safe for most people, and since it is used medicinally in very small amounts, this is also considered safe for most people. However, to be on the safe side, avoid larger amounts if you are pregnant or breastfeeding, or taking lithium or medicines changed by the liver (talk to your healthcare professional). Consumption of excessive amounts of black pepper can cause gastrointestinal irritation. Avoid large amounts if you have acid-peptic disease, stomach ulcers, ulcerative colitis, or diverticulitis.

30 Z. A. Damanhouri and A. Ahmad, "A Review on Therapeutic Potential of *Piper nigrum* L. (Black Pepper): The King of Spices," *Med Aromat Plants* 3:161, DOI:10.4172/2167-0412.1000161.

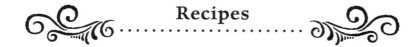

Recipes

BLACK PEPPER TEA

250 MILLILITRES (1 CUP) WATER

½ TEASPOON FRESHLY MILLED BLACK PEPPER.

Put the water and pepper in a pan and bring to boil. Simmer for four to five minutes. Remove from the heat and leave for ten minutes. Drink as required with a little honey, if liked. To improve the flavour, you can add a black teabag as you remove the pan from the heat, but don't forget to remove it when the desired strength is reached. For colds, you can add some fresh or powdered ginger to the pan as you simmer the pepper.

BLACK PEPPER COMPRESS

Prepare a double-strength **Black Pepper Tea** as above. Soak a clean cotton cloth in the hot infusion. Use this as hot as possible on the affected area (take care and do not burn yourself). Cover with a warm towel and leave for thirty minutes, and change the compress as it cools down. Use one to two times a day.

BLACK PEPPER MILK

250 MILLILITRES (1 CUP) MILK (SOYA OR ALMOND IS FINE)

1 PINCH FRESHLY MILLED BLACK PEPPER

1 PINCH TURMERIC POWDER

Warm the milk gently with the turmeric and black pepper; do not boil. This is an Ayurvedic remedy for treating coughs and colds.

. . . .

FIRE CIDER

1 TEASPOON BLACK PEPPERCORNS

5 GARLIC CLOVES, PEELED AND DICED

ZEST AND JUICE OF 2 LEMONS

1 SMALL ONION, PEELED AND DICED

3 CENTIMETRES GINGER, PEELED AND GRATED

1 TABLESPOON TURMERIC POWDER

1 TABLESPOON GRATED HORSERADISH

½ JALAPENO CHILLI PEPPER, DESEEDED AND CHOPPED

SPRIG OF FRESH ROSEMARY

CIDER VINEGAR

Put all the ingredients in a glass jar and add enough cider vinegar to cover all the ingredients well. Put on the lid and keep in a cool, dark place for four weeks, shaking daily. Strain off the liquid—this is your fire cider—and put it in a sterilised glass bottle. Store in the fridge. Take a teaspoon daily in the winter to ward off coughs and colds—if you like, you can take it in a cup of warm water with a teaspoon of honey. You can also use your fire cider externally as a warming muscle rub for aching muscles or rheumatism.

. . . .

BLACK PEPPER EXFOLIATING FACIAL SCRUB

½ TEASPOON BLACK PEPPER, FRESHLY GROUND

1 TABLESPOON YOGHURT (SOY YOGHURT IS FINE)

Blend together and use to very gently massage your skin in a circular motion for two or three minutes, being careful to avoid the sensitive eye area. Rinse off with lukewarm water and splash on cold water to seal the pores. Follow with a moisturiser. Do not use more than once a week, as it may irritate your skin if you do.

Caraway

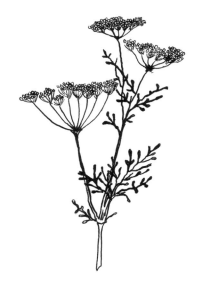

Carum carvi

PLANETARY RULER: Sun / Mercury

ELEMENT: Air

ASSOCIATED DEITIES: Sun goddesses, Saint Catherine

MAGICAL VIRTUES: Fidelity, love, memory, protection, retention

Caraway has been used since at least the Stone Age, with seed fragments found in food remains from this time. It is mentioned several times in the Bible, though this is actually a mistranslation; many versions still use the word *caraway* instead of *cumin*, which is actually what the peoples of the Bible would have known and used.

In England caraway is associated with the cycles of sowing and reaping. **Caraway Seed Cake** was traditionally served in English farmhouses after wheat sowing[31] and at the harvest suppers that were held for all the workers later on in the year. Special caraway cakes called **Cattern Cakes** were made on Saint Catherine's Day, November 25, and in Somerset farmers had special Cattern Pie shaped like a Catherine wheel (a pin wheel firework) and filled with mince, honey, and spices, washed down with "hot pot" made from warm beer, rum, and eggs. It is probable that Catherine was a Christianised version of an earlier goddess, represented as she is with a wheel, as were so many deities of the sun, fate, time, and the seasons. Wheels wrapped in straw and fired and rolled down hills were an ancient

---

31 Grieve, *A Modern Herbal*.

celebration of the sun and passage of the seasons. Use caraway in food, drink, and incenses at the vernal and autumnal equinoxes, or at times of beginning new projects or their coming to fruition.

Caraway seeds were widely believed to confer the gift of retention—any object that contained them could not be stolen or lost. Caraway dough was fed to chickens, doves, and pigeons to keep them from straying.[32] In fact, birds do love it, and this would certainly be an incentive to stay; it is still sometimes given to homing pigeons. You can use **Caraway Tea** or **Caraway Infused Oil** to anoint any objects or tools that you especially value to prevent their loss and bind them to you. Use **Caraway Seed Cake** as ritual food to bind a group together.

The power of retention even extended to spouses and lovers, and in folklore a cake or love potion given to a partner would keep them faithful and prevent them straying, while a few seeds placed in a wandering husband's pocket would prevent him being lured away. To ensure the fidelity of a bride and groom, guests would throw caraway seeds after the couple at the wedding. Today, hearth witches use caraway at handfastings to help couples to remain faithful, both in the ritual cup and in the cake. The rings may be consecrated with **Caraway Infused Oil** or incense. The couple may be served **Caraway Seed Cake**, but take care that no one else eats it!

However, because caraway has the power of retention, it is unlucky to give it away: there was an old saying that "you baked for me caraway bread but prepared yourself for tears."[33] You should definitely never give it to fairies, perhaps because caraway might be seen as binding them to the giver. The moss people, German woodland fairies who spin the moss for the forests, have a particular horror of it. Though they occasionally help humans, if they are thoughtlessly rewarded with gifts of caraway bread, they screech "Caraway bread, our death!"[34]

Caraway seeds were also believed to offer protection. In Germany parents placed a dish of caraway seeds beneath their childrens' beds to protect them not only from illness, but also from witches and fairies. It is said that witches themselves carried caraway seeds to protect them from an untimely death on the scaffold, while sprinkling caraway seeds on a loved one's coffin helps stop their soul being stolen by demons. To use caraway as a herb of protection, use **Caraway Tea** to cleanse the ritual working area or home; seal doors and

---

32 Ibid.

33 Cora Linn Daniels and C. M. Stevans, eds., *Encyclopædia of Superstitions, Folklore, and the Occult Sciences of the World*, volume I (University Press of the Pacific, 2003).

34 Jacob Grimm, *Deutsche Mythologie* (Wiesbaden, 2007).

windows with **Caraway Infused Oil** or **Caraway Tea**; and add to protection incenses. Sew caraway seed into a small white bag with white thread and hide it under the mattress of a child's crib or bed to keep the child free of illness and negativity. This also can be carried for protection by children and adults alike.

As a Mercury herb, caraway is associated with thought, memory, and communication. Use it in Mercury incense or in spells and rituals connected with communication, messages, and study. Carry a small yellow bag of caraway seeds to improve the memory.

CULINARY USES

In Shakespeare's *Henry IV*, Squire Shallow invites Falstaff to "a pippin and a dish of caraways," and the convention of serving apples with caraway continued to be a custom in England. At Trinity College, Cambridge, roast apples are still presented with a little saucer of caraway. Aromatic caraway seeds, with their mildly aniseed/ liquorice flavour, are often used in rye breads, biscuits and cakes, cheeses, soups, curries, dahl, biriyani, sauerkraut, paté, and sweets. Commercially, caraway is used as a flavouring for liqueurs such as kummel, aquavit, and schnapps. The leaves are also used for soups and stews, and the roots may be boiled and treated like cooked parsnips or carrots. Always buy the seeds whole and grind them just before use.

Please note that the so-called black caraway is actually from an entirely different plant, *Nigella sativa* L., and should not be confused with *Carum carvi*.

COSMETIC USES

The antioxidants in the caraway seeds can help protect your skin and hair. You can grind some caraway seeds, mix with honey, and apply to your skin as a face pack, massaging it gently, rinsing with warm water, and following with a moisturiser. You can also use this as a treat for your hair. Leave it on for thirty minutes, then shampoo as usual.

MEDICINAL USES

ACTIONS: anti-colitic, anti-inflammatory, antimicrobial, antioxidant, antispasmodic, aromatic, carminative, digestive, immunomodulatory, spasmolytic, stimulant

Caraway is related to dill, fennel, and anise and has been thought to have many of the same medicinal properties. They are all antispasmodic, carminative, and digestive herbs used to treat gas, bloating, and indigestion. In many parts of the world, a dish of caraway seeds is still served after a meal to help digestion and sweeten the breath. The Tudor Queen Elizabeth I had the following prescribed for wind: "Take ginger, cinnamon, galingale of each one ounce; aniseeds, caraway seeds, fennel seeds, of each half an ounce; mace and nut-megs two dram each; pound together and add one pound of white sugar. Use this powder after or before meat at any time. It comforteth the stomach, helpeth digestion, and expels wind greatly."[35] The whole seeds can be chewed raw or **Caraway Tea** taken.

Traditionally, caraway was a remedy for infant colic, and it is still used to flavour children's medicines. In America children were given caraway, fennel, and dill to chew during church services to stop them hiccupping, and they were dubbed the "three meetin'" seeds.

Caraway is also a good remedy for colds and chest congestion as it contains mild anti-histamines, antimicrobial compounds that help to relax the muscles that cause coughing spasms. Take a cup of **Caraway Tea** three times a day to ease the symptoms. You can also use double-strength **Caraway Tea** as a gargle for laryngitis.

Caraway is useful for skin irritations, boils, and rashes. They can be washed gently with **Caraway Tea** or you can powder the seeds in a grinder and mix with a little warm water and apply as a poultice. The latter will also help reduce bruises.

> CAUTION: Caraway is considered safe for most people in food amounts
> and for most people in medicinal amounts for up to eight weeks. To
> be on the safe side, medicinal amounts should be avoided during
> pregnancy and breastfeeding. It marginally lowers blood sugar, so if you
> are diabetic, monitor your levels carefully. Caraway should be avoided
> by those with hemochromatosis, as it increases iron absorption.

---

35   Quoted in Jane Lyle, A *Miscellany of Women's Wisdom* (Running Press, 1993).

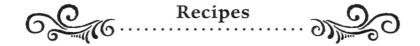

Recipes

CARAWAY TEA

1 TEASPOON SEEDS, LIGHTLY GROUND

250 MILLILITRES (1 CUP) BOILING WATER

Pour the boiling water over the seeds and infuse for fifteen minutes. Strain and take a cup up to three times daily.

CARAWAY SEED CAKE

110 GRAMS (½ CUP) BUTTER

170 GRAMS (¾ CUP) CASTOR (SUPERFINE) SUGAR

3 EGGS

2 TABLESPOONS COLD MILK

225 GRAMS (1¾ CUPS) PLAIN (BREAD) FLOUR

1 TEASPOON BAKING POWDER

50 GRAMS (6 TABLESPOONS) GROUND ALMONDS

1 TEASPOON CARAWAY SEEDS

Cream the butter and sugar together. Whisk the eggs with the milk, and gradually add this to the creamed butter and sugar. Fold in the flour and baking powder, then add the ground almonds and caraway seeds. Bake in a loaf tin lined with baking parchment for an hour at 160°C/325°F/gas mark 3.

CARAWAY INFUSED OIL

CARAWAY SEEDS

VEGETABLE OIL

Grind the dried seeds (use a pestle and mortar), but don't powder them. Put in a glass jar and cover with oil. Put on a sunny windowsill for three weeks, shaking daily. Strain the oil into a sterilised bottle. Store in a cool, dark place.

. . . .
Cattern Cakes

250 GRAMS (2 CUPS) SELF-RAISING FLOUR

¼ TEASPOON GROUND CINNAMON

60 GRAMS (1 CUP) CURRANTS

60 GRAMS (6½ TABLESPOONS) GROUND ALMONDS

2 TEASPOONS CARAWAY SEEDS

170 GRAMS (¾ CUP) CASTER (SUPERFINE) SUGAR

110 GRAMS (½ CUP) BUTTER, MELTED

1 MEDIUM EGG, BEATEN

MILK FOR BRUSHING

In a large mixing bowl, combine the flour, cinnamon, currants, ground almonds, caraway seeds, and sugar. Add the melted butter and beaten egg and mix well. On a floured board, roll the dough out to about 30 x 25 centimetres. Brush with milk and sprinkle on a little extra sugar and cinnamon. Roll the dough up like a Swiss roll and cut into 2 centimetre slices. Put them on a well-greased baking tray and bake at 200°C/400°F/gas mark 6 for ten to twelve minutes or until golden brown.

. . . .
Anti-bloating Tea

15 GRAMS (2½ TABLESPOONS) CARAWAY SEEDS

15 GRAMS (2½ TABLESPOONS) FENNEL SEEDS

15 GRAMS (2½ TABLESPOONS) ANISEED

Crush the seeds in a pestle and mortar. They can be stored for later use in an airtight jar or tin. To use, place 2 teaspoons of the seeds in a teapot, pour on 250 millilitres (1 cup) of boiling water, and infuse for ten minutes. Pour through a strainer into a cup and drink after meals if you have a tendency to bloat after eating.

. . . .
PROTECTION INCENSE

½ PART CARAWAY SEEDS

½ PART DRIED BASIL

¼ PART GROUND BLACK PEPPER

½ PART CINNAMON STICKS, CRUSHED

¼ PART GROUND CLOVES

¼ PART GINGER POWDER

½ PART DRIED ROSEMARY

½ PART DRIED THYME

Combine and burn on charcoal. If you have it, and wish to use it, you can add four parts frankincense resin, which will improve the burning quality and perfume, but this is optional and not necessary for the protective effect.

. . . . .

Cardamom

Elettaria spp. (native to India and Malasia)
Amomum spp. (native to Asia and Australia)

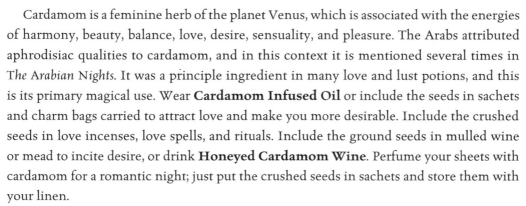

PLANETARY RULER: Venus

ELEMENT: Water

ASSOCIATED DEITIES: Erzulie, Hecate, Medea, Venus,
   Aphrodite, Three Graces

MAGICAL VIRTUES: Lust, love, harmony, balance, grace,
   attractiveness

Cardamom is a feminine herb of the planet Venus, which is associated with the energies of harmony, beauty, balance, love, desire, sensuality, and pleasure. The Arabs attributed aphrodisiac qualities to cardamom, and in this context it is mentioned several times in *The Arabian Nights*. It was a principle ingredient in many love and lust potions, and this is its primary magical use. Wear **Cardamom Infused Oil** or include the seeds in sachets and charm bags carried to attract love and make you more desirable. Include the crushed seeds in love incenses, love spells, and rituals. Include the ground seeds in mulled wine or mead to incite desire, or drink **Honeyed Cardamom Wine**. Perfume your sheets with cardamom for a romantic night; just put the crushed seeds in sachets and store them with your linen.

It is also a herb of friendship, of pleasure shared with others, and of harmony and grace. After all, the attendants of Aphrodite, the goddess of love, are the Three Graces—Thalia (Joy), Euphrosyne (Mirth), and Aglaea (Splendour)—who inspire poets and artists and bring joy, charm, and beauty to gods and men. They preside over all banquets, dances, and happy social events. To bring their grace into your life and to attract and be attractive, honour and invoke them at the full moon with three white candles anointed with **Cardamom Infused Oil**, for without love, friendship, fun, grace, beauty, and art, all striving is meaningless.

December 13 is a Swedish festival called "Little Yule." Though the Winter Solstice is the shortest day of the year, it is not the date of the earliest sunset, which occurs on Little Yule.[36] It is celebrated as the festival of Saint Lucy or Lucia, a mysterious and dangerous time in many parts of Europe, when witches were thought to be especially powerful. In preparation, the house was cleaned, all threshing, spinning, and weaving were finished, and candles were made. In Sweden today, on the day of the festival, the youngest daughter of the house rises before dawn, puts on a white dress and a crown of nine candles, and wakes the family with coffee and cakes seasoned with cardamom and saffron called *lussikatter* (**Lucy Cats**), said to refer to the devil's cats that Saint Lucy subdued. Whether an actual person called Saint Lucy/Lucia ever existed or not, the saint seems to have taken her mythology and characteristics from local Pagan deities, and as such is seen differently in different regions. It is likely that she originally derived from the Roman goddess Juno Lucina or Lucetia, the Mother of Light, who carried a tray and a lamp, bestowing the gifts of light, enlightenment, and sight, but in Scandinavia she seems to have taken on some attributes of the goddess Freya, who was associated with cats. Freya's special season was Yule, when she dispensed wealth and plenty. The traditional shape of the **Lucy Cat** rolls is a crossed shape with the arms rolled inwards in the form of a solar wheel.

CULINARY USES

There are two varieties of cardamom, the *Elettaria* grown in India, which is green or white, and the *Amomum* grown in China, which is black or dark brown. As a spice, cardamom is extremely versatile. You can buy it already ground, but the entire pod, opened to release the tiny black seeds inside for fresh grinding, is really the best way to use it.

Aromatic green cardamoms are used as flavouring agents in Indian cuisine, added to meat and vegetable dishes, breads, pickles, chutneys, desserts, sweets, and beverages. In Russia, Sweden, Norway, and parts of Germany, they are largely used for flavouring cakes and in the preparation of liqueurs.

---

36   Anna Franklin, *Yule, History, Lore and Celebration* (Lear Books, 2010).

The black cardamom has a full-bodied, smoky flavour and is used in savoury Chinese cuisine but never desserts and sweets.

Cardamom Coffee is popular in Arabic cultures. The seeds are ground and added to coffee grounds before brewing, or pods are steeped in the coffee itself.

COSMETIC USES

Cardamom is sweetly fragrant and often used in perfumery. However, for home use it is mainly employed to boost hair growth, combat dandruff, and protect the scalp from dryness and inflammation with its antimicrobial, anti-inflammatory, and antifungal actions. Massage your hair and scalp with **Cardamom Infused Oil** and leave on, covered with a warm towel, for thirty to sixty minutes. Wash and condition as usual.

MEDICINAL USES

ACTIONS: antimicrobial, anti-inflammatory, antifungal, antioxidant, stomachic, analgesic, carminative, expectorant

In ancient times cardamom was so valuable that it was largely relegated to medical purposes. It was one of the ingredients of the legendary nostrum Mithridate, said to have been invented by King Mithridates VI of Pontus (134 to 63 BCE), who used it to protect himself against poisons. The recipe is supposed to have been found by the Roman general Pompey, who took it back to Rome. Its semi-mythical status (and no doubt the cachet of its sixty expensive ingredients) made it one of the most sought-after remedies of the Middle Ages and Renaissance, and it was said to cure just about every ill under the sun.

Well, maybe not, but in traditional Indian medicine, Ayurveda, cardamom has a long-standing reputation for being an unparalleled stomachic. Consuming cardamom or integrating it into meals helps the stomach to better digest food. It has long been used as a remedy for digestive problems, including dyspepsia (indigestion), irritable bowel syndrome (IBS), and constipation.

Cardamom Tea can be drunk as a moderately effective analgesic (painkiller), especially for the treatment of moderate muscular pains and spasms. **Cardamom Infused Oil** may be used for the gentle massage of areas affected by arthritis or rheumatism.

Double-strength **Cardamom Tea** may be used as a topical rinse or medicated wash for the treatment of various skin disorders. **Cardamom Infused Oil** may be applied to dermatitis and fungal infections.

Double-strength **Cardamom Tea** may be gargled for bad breath, or you can simply chew the pods. The major active component of cardamom oil, cineole, is a powerful antiseptic known for killing the bacteria causing bad breath and other infections.

Those suffering from mouth ulcers or sore throats may also find a gargle of double-strength **Cardamom Tea** to be helpful.

CAUTION: Cardamom is considered safe for most people in food amounts. To be on the safe side, do not consume large amounts of cardamom if you are pregnant or breastfeeding. Only use small amounts of cardamom if you have gallstones, as large amounts can trigger gallstone colic.

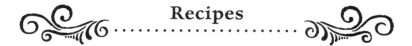

Recipes

Cardamom Tea

1 TEASPOON CARDAMOM SEEDS, CRUSHED

250 MILLILITRES (1 CUP) WATER

In a saucepan, bring the water up to a boil. Add the gently crushed cardamom seeds. Reduce the heat and simmer very gently fifteen to twenty minutes. Remove from heat and strain the liquid into a cup. Stir in a teaspoon of honey if desired.

Cardamom Coffee

250 MILLILITRES (1 CUP) WATER

1 TABLESPOON FINELY GROUND COFFEE

1 CARDAMOM POD, CRUSHED

In a pan, bring the water to a boil. Remove from heat and add coffee and cardamom. Return to the heat and bring to a boil. When it foams, remove it from the heat. Once again, put it back on the heat and bring to a boil, then strain it into a cup.

Honeyed Cardamom Wine

500 MILLILITRES (2 CUPS) RED WINE

500 MILLILITRES (2 CUPS) LUKEWARM WATER

4 TABLESPOONS HONEY, SLIGHTLY WARMED

1 CINNAMON STICK

¼ TEASPOON CARDAMOM, BLACK SEEDS ONLY, SLIGHTLY CRUSHED

Put the wine, water, and honey in a pot and add the spices. Cover and leave in a cool place for twenty-four hours. Strain and enjoy!

. . . .
Cardamom Infused Oil

1 TABLESPOON CARDAMOM SEEDS, LIGHTLY CRUSHED

500 MILLILITRES (2 CUPS) VEGETABLE OIL

In a double boiler, put in the seeds and cover with the vegetable oil. Simmer very gently, covered, for two hours. Turn off the heat and allow the oil to cool before straining.

. . . .
Aphrodisiac Incense

½ PART CARDAMOM SEEDS, CRUSHED

½ PART CINNAMON POWDER

¼ PART CLOVE, CRUSHED

½ PART CORIANDER SEEDS, CRUSHED

¼ PART GINGER POWDER

3 PARTS FRANKINCENSE RESIN

FEW DROPS CINNAMON ESSENTIAL OIL (OPTIONAL)

Blend together and burn on charcoal.

. . . .

LUCY CATS

400 MILLILITRES (1¾ CUPS) WHOLE MILK

½ TEASPOON SAFFRON

25 GRAMS (2 TABLESPOONS) DRIED YEAST

150 GRAMS (⅔ CUP) CASTER (SUPERFINE) SUGAR

200 GRAMS (¾ CUP PLUS 2 TABLESPOONS) PLAIN YOGURT

1 EGG, BEATEN

1 TEASPOON SALT

175 GRAMS (¾ CUP) BUTTER

800 GRAMS (6½ CUPS) PLAIN FLOUR

RAISINS

BEATEN EGG, FOR BRUSHING

Warm the milk slightly and put the saffron strands in. Leave to soak for about ten minutes. Sprinkle the yeast on with a teaspoon of the sugar, cover, and leave in a warm place to activate the yeast (when it goes frothy, it's activated). Blend in the rest of the sugar, then add the yoghurt, egg, and salt. Add the softened butter and flour and knead for ten minutes. Cover and leave the dough in a warm place until it has doubled in size (this will take about half an hour). Turn out the dough onto a floured board and knead again. Divide into twenty-five to thirty equal pieces. Using your hand, roll them out into "sausages." Put them on well-greased baking sheets in an S shape and pop a raisin into each of the two curves. Prove in a warm place for thirty minutes. Brush with a beaten egg and bake at 200°C/400°F/gas mark 6 for ten to twelve minutes or until browned.

Chilli/ Cayenne

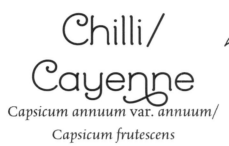

Capsicum annuum var. annuum/
Capsicum frutescens

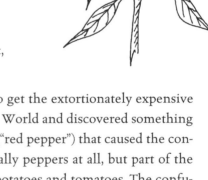

PLANETARY RULER: Mars

ELEMENT: Fire

ASSOCIATED DEITIES: Uchu, Alakshmi

MAGICAL VIRTUES: Shamanic travel, counter magic,
   protection, love, lust

Christopher Columbus set sail to find a new route to get the extortionately expensive black pepper cheaper, but instead he landed in the New World and discovered something just as good: chillies. It was his naming them pimiento ("red pepper") that caused the confusion that still exists with the name—they are not really peppers at all, but part of the Solanaceae or nightshade family, and so are related to potatoes and tomatoes. The confusion doesn't stop there; they are also called chile, chili, cayenne, paprika, and pimento.

Chillies are the only spice in this book with a New World origin. Chillies were called Uchu by the Incas and revered as a deity, one of the four brothers of a creation myth, and brother of the first Inca king. In his *Suma y narración de los Incas* ("Narrative of the Incas"), the Spaniard Juan de Betanzos included the story of the four Ayar brothers—Uchu, Manco, Cachi, and Auca—who with their four sisters/wives lived in a mountain cave called "Storehouse of Dawn." It had three windows, one of which looked out to the sky, one to the underworld, and one to the world of the living. The brothers and sisters left the cave in search of a suitable place to settle. Ayar Cache ("Salt"), was so powerful he could break mountains, so the siblings became afraid and sent him back to the cave, where he was walled up. The remaining siblings travelled through the Andes, planting seeds wherever they halted. When they reached the foot of the mountain Quirir-Manta, Ayar Uchu ("Hot Pepper")[37] became a stone shrine on the top of the mountain, where Inca youths went in order to be transformed into adults. Here the two brothers, Salt and Chilli Pepper, seem to represent shamanic opposite realms, one connected to the cave and earth, and the other connected with mountains and the sky.

Chilli peppers have certainly played their part in rituals of shamanic travel. The pre-Columbian tribes of Panama used chilli in combination with cocoa and other plants to enter into hallucinatory trance, travelling to the world above or the world below to negotiate with spirits on behalf of humankind.[38] In the Amazon chilli is sometimes added to the hallucinogenic medicines that shamans use for healing rituals and vision quests. The Aztecs also loved drinking *chilote*, a liqueur made of fermented agave pulp, chilli, and herbs, the basis of today's tequila and mezcal.

In Central and South America chillies were traditionally used in counter magic, protection rituals, and to drive out evil spirits. Sprinkled around the house, they were expected to repel malevolent demons and vampires, while burning them along with garlic and other pungent spices was intended to fumigate and purify the house. In Latin American countries they are also a popular counter-magical device to ward off or cure the effects of the evil eye. Strings of chilli peppers are hung up in the house or worn as a protective necklace.[39] Hang a string of dried chillies in your kitchen as a protective charm, or put a wreath of chillies and dried lemon slices on your front door. Add chilli powder to incenses of protection and banishing.

Chillies have long enjoyed a reputation as an aphrodisiac, as their fiery nature was thought to ignite the flames of passion. The Aztecs often mixed them with other aphrodisiac plants such as cocoa and vanilla. Share some **Chilli Hot Chocolate** or **Chilli Vodka** with a lover.

Add chilli powder to incenses of Mars and fire to increase their power.

---

37   http://cuzcoeats.com/the-myth-of-inca-origins-and-food, accessed 18 October 17.
38   http://www.chileplanet.eu/Origin-story.html, accessed 18 October 17.
39   Ibid.

CULINARY USES

Many villages in Central America are named after the type of chilli they grow, and special fiestas are celebrated in their honour. There are many hundreds of hybridized varieties of bell pepper and chilli in various shapes, colours, sizes, and degrees of heat. Most varieties are derived from the *annuum* species, though *C. frutescens* is also popular. The heat is identified in Scoville Heat Units, with bell peppers rating 0, cayenne 2,500–4,000, and habaneros up to 300,000!

Fresh chilli peppers can be used to make soups, stews, curries, chillies, spicy drinks, sauces, chutney, and pickles. Chilli powder and cayenne pepper are ground from the fruit of capsicums. Chilli powder is usually a blend of several types of chillies. It can be added to meat or vegetable dishes, pasta, and eggs.

MEDICINAL USES

ACTIONS: anti-inflammatory, analgesic, diuretic, stomachic, antianginal, antioxidant, detoxicant, antibiotic, sialagogue

Chilli pepper helps stimulate saliva, which is important for digestion as well as preventing bad breath. Use a **Chilli Gargle**.

The hot and spicy taste of chilli is due to a compound called capsaicin, which is a natural painkiller. Capsaicin depletes a neurotransmitter called substance P, which is responsible for sending pain signals to our brain. When applied topically to affected areas, this is very helpful in relieving pain in cases of osteoarthritis, rheumatoid arthritis, and fibromyalgia, as well as shingles, diabetic peripheral neuropathy, bursitis, and muscle and back pain. Rub the affected area with **Chilli Infused Oil** or **Chilli Salve**.

Eating chillies or drinking **Chilli Tea** aids in breaking up and moving congested mucus in cases of colds and flu. Chillies are also rich in vitamin C, which helps the immune system fight infections. Take some **Chilli Honey** or use a **Chilli Gargle** for laryngitis and sore throats. Eating hot peppers increases the flow of blood and loosens the secretions of mucus in the sinuses, thus relieving the congestion that causes sinus headaches.

CAUTION: Lotions and creams containing capsicum are thought to be safe for most adults when applied to the skin. However, side effects can include skin irritation, burning, and itching. Capsicum can also be extremely irritating to the eyes, nose, and throat. Never use around the eyes, mucous membranes, or on sensitive or broken skin. Do not use on children. Eating chillies is safe for most people, but very hot chillies can cause stomach irritation and upset, sweating, flushing, and a runny nose. Very large doses over a period of time may cause more serious side effects. Do not use if you are breastfeeding, and stay on the safe side and don't use more than small culinary amounts if you are pregnant. Stop using chillies at least two weeks before a scheduled surgery. Take care if you take anticlotting medications including aspirin, as capsicum may increase the effect. Avoid if you take theophylline.

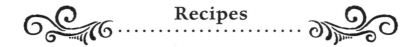

Recipes

Chilli Honey

2 TEASPOONS LEMON JUICE

1 TABLESPOON HONEY

PINCH OF CHILLI POWDER

Simply combine the ingredients and take a teaspoonful as required.

Chilli Hot Chocolate

750 MILLILITRES (3 CUPS) MILK

½ VANILLA POD

1 CINNAMON STICK

1 RED CHILLI, DESEEDED

2 TEASPOONS COCOA POWDER

130 GRAMS (½ CUP) DARK CHOCOLATE, GRATED

Put the milk, vanilla pod, cinnamon stick, and chilli in a saucepan over a medium heat until boiling. Remove from the heat and leave for ten minutes to infuse. Strain the liquid into a clean pan over a medium heat (don't boil), and add the cocoa powder and chocolate, stirring until smooth. If you wish, serve topped with whipped cream.

Chilli Gargle

125 MILLILITRES (½ CUP) WATER

1 TABLESPOON LEMON JUICE

1 TEASPOON SALT

PINCH CHILLI POWDER

Mix the ingredients and use it as a gargle several times a day to aid a sore throat. For laryngitis, substitute honey for the salt.

. . . .
Chilli Infused Oil

10-12 FRESH CHILLI PEPPERS

500 MILLILITRES (2 CUPS) VEGETABLE OIL

Put the chillies and oil in a food processor or liquidiser and whizz up. Put the mixture in a glass jar and leave in a cool, dark place for ten days. Strain the liquid through fine muslin into a sterilised bottle. Apply directly to painful joints. Wash your hands afterwards and avoid broken skin or touching the eye area.

. . . .
Chilli Salve

4 FRESH CHILLIES, CHOPPED

200 MILLILITRES (¾ CUP) VEGETABLE OIL

1 TABLESPOON BEESWAX

Put the chillies and oil in a double boiler and simmer for about fifty minutes. Strain out the chillies and return the oil to the pan. Add the beeswax and stir until it has melted. Pour into warmed, sterilised glass jars. Apply directly to your painful joints. Do not use on broken skin. Wash your hands afterwards and avoid touching the eye area.

. . . .
Chilli Tea

1 TEASPOON GROUND CHILLI PEPPER

250 MILLILITRES (1 CUP) WATER

Pour the boiling water over the chilli pepper and infuse for ten minutes before drinking.

. . . .
Banishing Incense

½ PART DRIED BASIL

¼ PART BLACK PEPPER, GROUND

¼ PART CHILLI POWDER

½ PART CLOVE, CRUSHED

¼ PART DILL SEEDS, CRUSHED

½ PART GARLIC POWDER OR GARLIC SALT

½ PART LEMON PEEL, CHOPPED

Combine and burn on charcoal. You can add four parts of frankincense resin if you have it, but this is not necessary to obtain the magical effect.

. . . .
Chilli Vodka

4 CHILLIES

500 MILLILITRES (2 CUPS) VODKA

Prick the chillies and put them in a bottle and top up with the vodka. Leave to infuse for two weeks, then strain off the vodka into a clean bottle.

. . . . .

Cinnamon

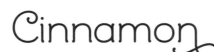

Cinnamonum verum syn.
Cinnamonum zeylanicum

PLANETARY RULER: Sun

ELEMENT: Fire

ASSOCIATED DEITIES: Helios, Ra, Apollo, Aphrodite,
Venus, Dionysus, Aesculapius

MAGICAL VIRTUES: Warming, energising, protection,
healing, regeneration, divination, love, passion

Cinnamon generally refers to "true" cinnamon or Ceylon cinnamon (*Cinnamonum verum* syn. *Cinnamonum zeylanicum*), though this is sometimes adulterated with (or substituted by) cassia or Chinese cinnamon (*Cinnamonum cassia*) from a different but related tree grown in China, which is not only cheaper but rougher and hotter in taste. In fact, around 250 species of cinnamon have been identified, and the spice purchased in shops may be a combination of several varieties.

The ancients thought of cinnamon as a mystical plant with fabulous origins. According to Theophrastus, it only grew in deep glens guarded by deadly snakes so that those who ventured there to collect it risked their lives, covering their hands and feet in a bid to protect themselves from the vipers.[40] Once harvested, they divided it into three equal portions, leaving one behind as an offering to the sun, whose plant it was, which spontaneously

---

40 Theophrastus, *Enquiry into Plants.*

burst into flames as the sun accepted it.[41] Herodotus wrote that cinnamon grew in the lands where the wild god Dionysus was raised and where large birds built their nests from cinnamon sticks.[42] These were called spice birds, and Pliny said they belonged to a species of phoenix, a mythical bird associated with the sun that rises reborn from the ashes of its own funeral pyre, a symbol of renewal, rebirth, and regeneration. In other stories fennel, cinnamon, and spikenard were used to build the funeral pyre of the phoenix; in others the phoenix produces no dung except a worm that turns into cinnamon.

Cinnamon, ruled by the sun and the element of fire, is certainly filled with solar energies, which are warming, energising, protective, healing, and facilitate divination. It may be used in incenses, potions, sachets, charm bags, rituals, and spells for all these purposes. Cinnamon is intimately connected in myth with the regeneration of the phoenix, a solar symbol, and therefore with the rebirth of the sun itself. This means it comes into its own at Yule, when we add it to the ritual fire that burns away the old and gives birth to the new. This is also a ritual that you can use when you need to end one cycle or situation and begin a new one—burn away a symbol or token of the past on a small fire that includes cinnamon sticks, and watch the flame of new beginnings arise.

The fantastical tales of cinnamon's origins meant that cinnamon was a prized and expensive commodity in the ancient world. In the first century CE the Roman historian Pliny the Elder wrote that a pound of cinnamon was fifteen times the value of silver. This meant it was a gesture of supreme extravagance when the emperor Nero ordered an entire year's worth of cinnamon imports to be gathered from around the Roman Empire to burn on his wife Poppaea Sabina's funeral pyre in 65 CE, to signify his remorse at having killed her by kicking her in the stomach in a fit of temper.[43]

Cinnamon is one of the oldest recorded aromatic plants, mentioned in the Old Testament as one of the spices given to Solomon by the Queen of Sheba. Its use was essentially for spiritual purposes, employed in anointing oils and incenses. In the Bible, Jehovah ordered Moses to make a holy ointment with olive oil, five hundred units of myrrh and cassia, and half as much of sweet cinnamon and calamus in order to anoint the sanctuary and its furnishings and priests.[44] At the Egyptian temple of Edfu, a recipe for incense was found dating to 1500 BCE, using the ingredient *kainamaa*, identified as cinnamon.[45] Egyp-

---

41 Pliny the Elder, *The Natural History*.
42 Herodotus, *The History of Herodotus*.
43 Brunton-Seal and Seal, *Kitchen Medicine*, and Swain, *The Lore of Spices*.
44 Exodus 30.
45 Swain, *The Lore of Spices*.

tian recipes for **Kyphi**, an aromatic used for burning, have included cinnamon and cassia from Hellenistic times onwards.

Today, modern witches use cinnamon in incenses for much the same reasons—it resonates with the energy of the sun, it raises magical vibration, and it creates a peaceful energy. It is useful for rituals of healing and divination. **Cinnamon Tea** may be taken to attune and clear the mind beforehand.

Warm, spicy cinnamon is also a herb of love and passion. In the Old Testament there are several verses about the enticing nature of cinnamon, such as this one from Proverbs: "I have perfumed my bed with myrrh, aloes and cinnamon. Come, let us take our fill of love till morning."[46] It was commonly thought of as an aphrodisiac. In England newlyweds used to be given a posset for the marriage bed of wine, sugar, milk, egg yolk, sugar, cinnamon and nutmeg to help the performance along.[47] In sexual or Tantric magic, **Cinnamon Infused Oil**, used to anoint the body, stimulates male passion with sun energy. Cinnamon may be mixed with other herbs and spices in the ritual cup shared between a couple engaged in such practices, in the Great Rite, or, indeed, in the handfasting cup. Cinnamon and **Cinnamon Infused Oil** can be used in love spells and to make charms to draw love, happiness, and money.

CULINARY USES

Cinnamon is used to flavour a variety of foods, from sweets and desserts to drinks, casseroles, and curries. The ground spice is used in cakes, biscuits, on baked apples, custards, and for the nursery tea of cinnamon toast where it is combined with butter and sugar and spread on hot toast. Add a stick of cinnamon to rice when it is boiling to add an interesting depth of flavour. It is wonderful in mulled wine and punches. The powder keeps about a year in a dark glass jar, after which it loses potency and should be replaced.

COSMETIC USES

Cinnamon is used in some proprietary beauty products, shampoos, and perfumes, not just for its luscious scent, but also for its many benefits. It contains antioxidants and nutrients that stimulate hair growth, plump the skin, stimulate collagen growth, and tighten loose skin. It has antibiotic and antimicrobial effects that protect skin from irritation and infection. Try combining a teaspoon of powdered cinnamon with a tablespoon of honey to

---

46 Proverbs 7, 17–18.
47 Brunton-Seal and Seal, *Kitchen Medicine*.

make a face mask, spread on, leave for fifteen minutes, and rinse off with warm water. Add **Cinnamon Tea** to the bath for a warming and skin-tightening effect.

For a cinnamon hair treatment, combine a teaspoon of cinnamon powder with a slightly warmed 200 millilitres of olive oil and work into your scalp and hair. Cover with a warm towel and leave for thirty minutes, then shampoo and condition as usual.

MEDICINAL USES

ACTIONS: carminative, astringent, anti-inflammatory, anti-emetic, antimicrobial, warming, diaphoretic, circulatory stimulant

Cinnamon was much valued as a medicinal plant in the ancient world and has been part of the Chinese pharmacopoeia since the Shen Nung period, around 2800 BCE. In England the Venerable Bede (672–735 CE) said that cinnamon and cassia were "very effective in curing disorders of the guts,"[48] while the twelfth-century abbess and herbalist Hildegard von Bingen called it the "universal spice for sinuses" and a treatment for colds and flu.[49]

Cinnamon has been used to alleviate gastrointestinal problems in both Eastern and Western medicine for centuries. The tannins in cinnamon make it slightly astringent and therefore good for nausea and diarrhoea. **Cinnamon Tea** with honey and lemon can help the nausea and diarrhoea caused by gastric infections.[50] It is also useful for those who have a weak digestion and a poor appetite.[51] The German Commission E (equivalent of the FDA) endorses the use of cinnamon for indigestion, bloating, and flatulence.[52] To alleviate digestive symptoms, take a cup of **Cinnamon Tea** or add cinnamon to food. If you suffer from constipation, larger amounts of cinnamon have a laxative effect without the flatulence and intestinal cramping that can accompany proprietary laxatives.

Because cinnamon lowers inflammation, it can be beneficial in pain management, with studies showing that cinnamon helps to relieve arthritis, muscle soreness, and menstrual cramps. It also contains eugenol, a natural anaesthetic that helps relieve pain,[53] so topical applications of cinnamon in the form of a cinnamon compress (dip a cloth in **Cinnamon Tea**), **Cinnamon Infused Oil**, or **Cinnamon Salve** may be helpful.

---

48   Quoted in Brunton-Seal and Seal, *Kitchen Medicine.*
49   Quoted in Castleman, *The New Healing Herbs.*
50   Chown and Walker, *The Handmade Apothecary.*
51   Bartram, *Bartram's Encyclopaedia of Herbal Medicine.*
52   Castleman, *The New Healing Herbs.*
53   Ibid.

Cinnamon is a drying herb that helps to dry and clear mucus from the sinuses and lungs in cases of coughs and colds. You can just chew on a cinnamon stick, use **Cinnamon Electuary**, suck **Cinnamon Cough Drops**, or drink **Cinnamon Tea**. It helps fight off winter infections, and older or vulnerable people may wish to include cinnamon in their diets as a preventative.

Cinnamon is a powerful antiseptic. It kills many decay- and disease-causing bacteria, fungi, and viruses. Try sprinkling some cinnamon powder on cuts and small wounds after they have been thoroughly washed. Cinnamon has been traditionally used as a **Tooth Powder**.[54] It has been shown to be protective against the oral bacteria that can cause bad breath, tooth decay, cavities, and mouth infections, naturally combatting bacteria in the mouth and acting like a natural antibacterial treatment.[55]

Cinnamon helps to reduce high cholesterol. Compounds in cinnamon are able to help reduce levels of total cholesterol, LDL ("bad") cholesterol, and triglycerides, while HDL ("good") cholesterol remains stable. Cinnamon has also been shown to reduce high blood pressure, which is another threat for causing heart disease or a stroke. Add cinnamon to meals, take **Cinnamon Tea**, or have some **Cinnamon Milk** each day.

> CAUTION: Cinnamon is considered safe for most people, though
> continued use can occasionally irritate the mouth in some people,
> and skin applications may cause redness and irritation. It should
> not be used in very large amounts by people with liver problems,
> diabetics (it lowers blood sugar) unless levels are carefully monitored,
> women who are pregnant or breastfeeding, or by young children.

54 V. Jakhetia, R. Patel, P. Khatri, et al., "Cinnamon: A Pharmacological Review," *Journal of Advanced Scientific Research* 1, no. 2 (2010).

55 Pasupuleti Visweswara Rao and Siew Hua Gan, "Cinnamon: A Multifaceted Medicinal Plant," *Evidence-Based Complementary and Alternative Medicine*, vol. 2014, article ID 642942, 12 pages, 2014. https://doi.org/10.1155/2014/642942.

Recipes

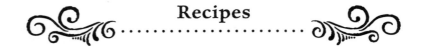

Cinnamon Milk

250 MILLILITRES (1 CUP) WARM MILK (SOYA, ALMOND, ETC. IS FINE)

¼ TEASPOON CINNAMON POWDER

1 TEASPOON HONEY (OPTIONAL)

2 DROPS VANILLA EXTRACT

Combine and drink.

Cinnamon Tea

1 CINNAMON STICK

250 MILLILITRES (1 CUP) WATER

Put the ingredients in a pan and boil for fifteen minutes. Remove from the heat and let stand for ten minutes. Strain and drink.

Cinnamon Electuary

Combine 4 teaspoons powdered cinnamon in a jar of honey. There is no need to strain this afterwards.

Cinnamon Infused Oil

6 CINNAMON STICKS, CRUSHED

500 MILLILITRES (2 CUPS) VEGETABLE OIL

In a double boiler, put in the crushed cinnamon sticks and cover with oil. Simmer very gently, covered, for two hours. Turn off the heat and allow the oil to cool before straining.

. . . .
Cinnamon Salve

CINNAMON INFUSED OIL (SEE PAGE 80)

BEESWAX

Gently warm the oil and add beeswax, allowing 2 tablespoons of grated beeswax to 500 millilitres of infused oil after the herbal material has been strained off. Remove from the heat and pour into shallow glass jars to set.

. . . .
Cinnamon Tooth Powder

1 TABLESPOON BICARBONATE OF SODA (BAKING SODA)

1 TABLESPOON SALT

2 TEASPOONS CINNAMON

Mix all ingredients together and store in an airtight container. Dip your damp toothbrush in it and brush. You can make this into toothpaste by adding a few drops of food-grade vegetable glycerine.

. . . .
Cinnamon Cough Drops

2 TABLESPOONS ROSE WATER

2 TEASPOONS GUM ARABIC

6 TABLESPOONS CASTER (SUPERFINE) SUGAR

6 TABLESPOONS CINNAMON POWDER

Warm the rose water and dissolve the gum Arabic in it. Mix together equal amounts of cinnamon and caster (superfine) sugar, and work this into the gum paste. Keep adding some until it becomes quite solid. You can shape this into little pastilles and leave them on greaseproof paper to dry. Roll in powdered sugar and store in an airtight container.

. . . .

KYPHI INCENSE

Part 1

    ½ PART HONEY

    ¼ PART RED WINE

    2 PARTS JUNIPER BERRIES

Part 2

    4 PARTS MYRRH RESIN

    2 PARTS FRANKINCENSE

    1 PART PINE RESIN

    ½ PART CARDAMOM

    ½ PART CASSIA

    1 PART CINNAMON STICKS, POUNDED

    PINCH SAFFRON

    ½ PART DRIED MINT LEAVES

Combine the part 1 ingredients of crushed juniper berries with the honey and wine. Put this in an airtight container with a lid and set it aside for seven days. When seven days have elapsed, combine all the part 2 ingredients together and then stir in the part 1 mixture well. To use, burn small amounts on charcoal.

Clove

Syzygium aromaticum
syn. *Carophyllus aromaticus /*
Eugenia aromatic /
E. caryophyllata/
E. a caryophyllus

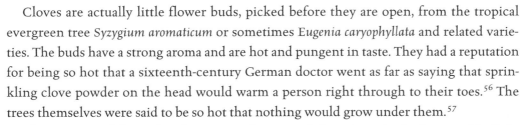

PLANETARY RULER: Sun, Jupiter

ELEMENT: Fire

ASSOCIATED DEITIES: None

MAGICAL VIRTUES: Protection, banishing, exorcism, love,
   prosperity, astral travel

Cloves are actually little flower buds, picked before they are open, from the tropical evergreen tree *Syzygium aromaticum* or sometimes *Eugenia caryophyllata* and related varieties. The buds have a strong aroma and are hot and pungent in taste. They had a reputation for being so hot that a sixteenth-century German doctor went as far as saying that sprinkling clove powder on the head would warm a person right through to their toes.[56] The trees themselves were said to be so hot that nothing would grow under them.[57]

The Latin word for *nail* is the origin of our word *clove* since the buds resemble little nails, and one of the primary uses of cloves in magic is in "nailing" or stopping the effects

---

56   Swain, *The Lore of Spices.*
57   Ibid.

of the evil eye, and this is a very widespread belief throughout the world. In Greece, for example, cloves are held and the fingers of one hand pointed at the person causing the evil eye while saying "Nails to your eyes!"[58] Amongst the Jews of the Iberian Peninsula, cloves were waved over the head of the affected with the words "I recite this formula. I recite the ritual formula to my daughter; she does not cause harm nor should harm be done to her. With these cloves may she find the remedy," after which the cloves were burned in hot coals, and when they exploded it was imagined that the eyes of whoever cast the evil eye would explode with them.[59] Further afield, a ceremony was recorded of an exorcism on the banks of the Ganges in the 1990s, in which a young woman who had had a miscarriage and thought she might have been cursed by a neighbour was touched by an exorcist with a clove to take out the evil. He touched her head with the clove, casting out the demon in the name of the Goddess. He then touched the clove to her stomach, again casting out any problems, saying he was taking out the witchcraft. He then placed the clove into the mouth of a live fish and released it into the river while repeating "I will never come again."[60]

Cloves can be employed in spells and rituals to stop or "nail" malicious magic against you. Light a white candle and take five cloves. Pass them three times over your head, then ignite each one in the flame (use tongs), saying, "Here I remove the evil eye and the evil speech; all manner of evil I cast into the flame." If one pops, you can be sure that the magic has hit its target. Allow the clove smoke to purify you. Put any remaining clove pieces on a dish and cast them into running water.

There is an old belief that children can be preserved from harm and illness by wearing a necklace of clove buds,[61] while a necklace of cloves strung on a red thread was hung above a baby's crib for protection. You can follow this tradition and string cloves on thread or put seven cloves in a white charm bag hung above a child's bed.

In Greece cloves are also used in a pre-wedding ritual to protect the bride. Cloves are soaked in water overnight and then the bride's mother takes a needle and thread and threads a gold coin and three cloves. All the other women then thread cloves to make a necklace for the bride, singing and invoking protection for her. The bride will keep the necklace safely put away and pass it on to her daughter. The guests at this ceremony also make protective clove amulets for themselves, and wrapped cloves are offered in little

---

58   Petropoulos, *Greek Magic, Ancient, Medieval and Modern.*
59   Levy and Levy Zumwalt, *Ritual Medical Lore of Sephardic Women.*
60   Ariel Glucklich, *The End of Magic* (Oxford University Press, New York), 1997.
61   Folkard, *Plant Lore, Legends, and Lyrics.*

packets to those invited to the ritual of making up the marriage bed.[62] This is a nice custom to introduce to handfastings, and the women of the clan can get together beforehand to perform such magic.

Old herbals account clove to be an aphrodisiac, suggesting that men could regain their potency by drinking sweet milk and crushed cloves.[63] Clove was a prime ingredient of many love potions, commonly used in love philtres or carried in the pocket to attract a lover. Simply infuse cloves into wine, mead, or alcoholic apple cider to enjoy its effects. Cloves may be added to the ritual cup or the incense for handfastings.

Cloves are also associated with prosperity and can be added to money drawing and good luck charm bags. **Clove Infused Oil** can be used to anoint a green candle in a prosperity spell.

Lightly ground cloves are a lovely incense ingredient, adding warmth and a depth of perfume to the formula. They may be added to incenses of the sun, Jupiter, fire, love, prosperity, and protection. They can also be used in incenses designed to aid astral travel, or **Clove Tea** may be taken for this purpose.

CULINARY USES

Cloves can be used whole or ground, but they have a very strong, pungent taste and aroma, so should be used sparingly—a little goes a long way, and too much is unpleasant and overpowering. Whole cloves are best removed from a dish before serving.

Cloves are used in the cuisines of Asia, Africa, the Middle East, and South and Central America, and they have been known and used in Western Europe for over a thousand years. They lend flavour to meat dishes, curries, side dishes, casseroles, and stews, and are used in marinades and condiments such as Worcestershire sauce. They are popular in desserts, often paired with cinnamon and nutmeg, and work especially well with fruit such as apples, pears, and pumpkin. Cloves are an essential component of some beverages such as mulled wine and egg nog, and they are a common element in many spice blends such as pumpkin pie spice, garam marsala, Chinese five spice, and curry powder.

COSMETIC USES

Clove is a natural antiseptic and can be used to combat spots and breakouts. Combine ground cloves with honey and apply to spots. Leave for fifteen minutes and rinse off with warm water.

---

62   Petropoulos, *Greek Magic, Ancient, Medieval and Modern.*
63   Swain, *The Lore of Spices.*

MEDICINAL USES

ACTIONS: antiseptic, expectorant, anaesthetic, antioxidant, rubefacient

A clove can be your mouth's best friend! Traditional Chinese medicine and Ayurveda both used cloves for toothache. Eugenol, one of the active ingredients in cloves, is an anaesthetic, and this is why clove oil is still used by some dentists as well as being included in over-the-counter toothache remedies. You can apply clove oil to the affected tooth (clove essential oil should be used very sparingly and rarely) or just put a clove in contact with the tooth. Be aware that this is an emergency measure and you should consult a dentist as soon as possible, as continued use will irritate the gum tissue. Never use this method for children, who are more sensitive to the chemicals in cloves and can suffer serious side effects. Cloves are also useful for gum diseases like gingivitis, periodontitis, and oral thrush, controlling the growth of oral pathogens and having powerful antifungal properties—just rinse with **Clove Tea**. Furthermore, a rinse with cloves will also stop bad breath. In the third century BCE, a Chinese leader in the Han Dynasty required those who addressed him to chew cloves to freshen their breath. They would have to take a clove from a proffered bowl and suck on it while they addressed the emperor.[64]

Cloves can help you clear a respiratory infection. They work as an expectorant, loosening mucus in the throat and oesophagus. Try **Clove and Cinnamon Tea** or rub **Clove and Coconut Balm** or **Clove Infused Oil** onto your chest. Applied to the skin, the volatile oils in clove function as a rubefacient, meaning that it slightly irritates the skin and expands the blood vessels, increasing the flow of blood to the surface. This is helpful for arthritis and sore muscles, used either as a **Clove Compress** or using **Clove Tea** in a hot bath or applying **Clove and Coconut Balm** or **Clove Infused Oil** to the affected area. Clove is also a topical anaesthetic, dulling pain, while the eugenol it contains is a powerful anti-inflammatory.

> CAUTION: Cloves are considered safe for most people when consumed in food amounts or when applied to the skin. However, frequent and repeated application of clove essential oil or clove buds to the tissues of the mouth can sometimes cause damage and should *never* be used on children. Stay on the safe side and avoid larger amounts of clove if you are pregnant or breastfeeding, have a bleeding disorder, and for three weeks before surgery, as clove oil contains a chemical called eugenol that slows blood clotting.

---

64   Swain, *The Lore of Spices.*

Recipes

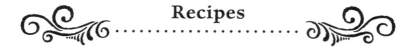

Clove Infused Oil

50 GRAMS (½ CUP) FRESHLY GROUND CLOVES

300 MILLILITRES (1½ CUPS) VEGETABLE OIL

Put the cloves and oil in a double boiler and simmer very gently for two hours. Strain into a clean bottle, label, and store in a cool, dark place.

Clove Tea

3 CLOVES

250 MILLILITRES (1 CUP) WATER

Put in a pan and simmer for twenty minutes. Remove from the heat and leave to stand for another ten minutes. Strain and drink with a little honey.

Clove and Cinnamon Tea

2 CLOVES, CRUSHED

1 STICK OF CINNAMON, CRUSHED

250 MILLILITRES (1 CUP) WATER

Put everything in a pan and simmer for twenty minutes. Remove from the heat and leave to stand for another ten minutes. Strain and drink with a little honey.

Clove Compress

For a compress, prepare a clean cotton cloth and soak it in hot clove tea. Use this as hot as possible on the affected area (take care and do not burn yourself). Cover with a warm towel and leave for thirty minutes. Change the compress as it cools down. Use one to two times a day.

· · · · · · · · · · · · · · · · ·
Clove and Coconut Balm

200 GRAMS (1 CUP) SOLID COCONUT OIL

30 GRAMS (½ CUP) CLOVES, FRESHLY GROUND

In a double boiler, simmer together for two hours. Strain through muslin into a shallow jar. Rub onto painful joints and muscles.

· · · · · · · · · · · ·
Clove Electuary

6 CLOVES

300 MILLILITRES (1¼ CUPS) RUNNY HONEY, WARMED

Combine and leave for three days. Strain off the cloves and take a teaspoon as needed. Cloves dull the pain, and the honey soothes.

· · · · · · · · · · · · · · · · · ·
Clove and Ginger Metheglin

2 KILOS (6 CUPS) HONEY

4 LITRES (17 CUPS) WATER

15 GRAMS (2½ TABLESPOONS) GINGER

2 CLOVES

YEAST

30 GRAMS (8 TABLESPOONS) DRIED HOPS

Boil the honey, 2 litres of water, ginger, and cloves until the liquid is reduced by one quarter. Skim off the scum and cool to lukewarm. Add the yeast. Boil the hops in 2 litres of water. Cool to lukewarm and add to the rest. Pour into a plastic brewing bin, fit the lid, and leave to stand for six weeks. Strain into a demijohn and fit an airlock. After six months you can syphon off your metheglin into bottles.

· · · · ·

. . . .
Abundance Incense

½ PART CRUSHED CLOVES

½ PART CINNAMON BARK

¼ PART NUTMEG POWDER

¼ PART DRIED BASIL

FEW DROPS CINNAMON ESSENTIAL OIL (OPTIONAL)

2 PARTS FRANKINCENSE (OPTIONAL)

Blend at the waxing moon and burn on charcoal.

Coriander

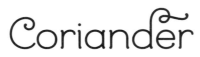

Coriandrum sativum

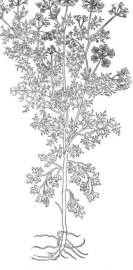

PLANETARY RULER: Mars

ELEMENT: Fire

ASSOCIATED DEITIES: Aphrodite, Venus, Ariadne, Ana, Anatu, Anahita

MAGICAL VIRTUES: Love, passion, peace, protection

In Britain both the fruit (called seeds) and fresh leaves are called coriander, while in the United States the seeds keep the name coriander, but the leaves take the Spanish name for the plant, cilantro, owing to their extensive use in Mexican cookery. The word *coriander* is believed to be derived from the Greek word *koris*, which means "a bedbug,"[65] and this is thought to refer to the strong scent of the leaves caused by the aldehydic components of the essential oil present, which some people hate and others, like me, love. It is certainly named after a bug in several languages, but the earliest attested form of the word is the Mycenaean Greek written in Linear B syllabic script, reconstructed as *koriadnon* or *koriandron*.[66] *Ari* means "most" and *adnos* means "holy," and this is also the derivation of Ariadne's name, the Minoan goddess of the labyrinth, so there may be a lost legend here connecting the two—or, at least, coriander must have been considered a very holy herb used in ancient Crete. Coriander is certainly associated with the Phoenician/Canaanite goddess

65 Swain, *The Lore of Spices.*

66 John Chadwick, *The Mycenaean World* (Cambridge University Press, 1976).

Ana (Anatu/Anahita), titled Virgin, Mother of Nations, or She Who Kills and Resurrects, the consort of Ba'al who wore horns and carried a moon disc and wore coriander perfume. Coriander was much valued as a perfume in the ancient world.[67]

Pliny wrote that fresh coriander was believed to be an aphrodisiac, adding that some thought it beneficial to place coriander beneath the pillow before sunrise.[68] There is some evidence that coriander seeds were placed in Egyptian tombs as a symbol of eternal love and enduring passion.[69] Similarly, in Chinese tradition it was considered both a herb of immortality and an aphrodisiac.[70] It is mentioned several times in *The Arabian Nights* as arousing sexual desires, and in Europe in the Middle Ages and Renaissance it was considered to provoke lust and love and added to love potions. The seeds were put into the popular drink **Hippocras**, which was commonly drunk at Tudor weddings. Culpeper designated coriander as "hot in the first degree," a herb of Mars,[71] and rather than romantic gentle love and friendship, it is used in spells of lust and passion and added to love charms and incenses. Coriander also can be used to anoint the candles used in love magic, be included in the ritual cup at handfastings and Great Rite celebrations, and be added to the handfasting cake.

You can throw coriander seeds instead of confetti at handfastings; indeed, coriander seeds may have been the original confetti. The fruits used to be made into the sweets called *confits*, coated in white or pink sugar. These were thrown into the crowds from the backs of carnival wagons. However, eventually this was thought to be wasteful, and they were replaced by bits of coloured paper but kept their original name "confetti."[72]

The passionate nature of coriander helps bring sweetness and hope back into life after suffering personal loss or a broken heart. Use **Coriander Flower Essence** or **Coriander Leaf Tea** when you feel disconnected from other people, life, or the universe and your spiritual connections.

---

67   John Chadwick, *The Mycenaean World* (Cambridge University Press, 1976).
68   Pliny the Elder, *The Natural History*.
69   Spices of Life in Ancient Egypt, http://www.history.com/news/hungry-history /spices-of-life-in-ancient-egypt, accessed 26 September 17.
70   Brunton-Seal and Seal, *Kitchen Medicine*.
71   *Culpeper's Complete Herbal*.
72   Swain, *The Lore of Spices*.

CULINARY USES

The Romans were very fond of coriander. They used it in a sophisticated seasoning mixture that included wild celery, coriander, mint, onion, pennyroyal, rue, savory, and thyme.

Coriander (cilantro) leaves are best used fresh to preserve the volatile oils responsible for the taste and aroma. They can be chopped and sprinkled on curries, stir fries, added to salsas, and so on. Try making a coriander pesto instead of a basil one for a taste sensation, or add to your juicer to benefit from coriander leaf's antioxidants. The dried seeds are available whole or ground, but for best results, buy them whole and crush them lightly in a pestle and mortar just before use. They flavour curries, breads, sauces, soups, stews, pastries, and sweets and are used commercially to flavour gin.

COSMETIC USES

Coriander leaf contains antioxidants to combat damaging free radicals, plus minerals and vitamins that help in the battle against wrinkles and sagging skin. They also have a cooling, antiseptic, detoxifying, and soothing action. To benefit, try a face mask from a paste of fresh coriander leaves mixed with a little honey. Apply to the face, leave twenty minutes, and rinse off with warm water.

A hair rinse made from **Coriander Leaf Tea** will promote new hair growth.

MEDICINAL USES

ACTIONS: anaesthetic, anti-arthritic, antibacterial, antifungal, anti-inflammatory, antioxidant, antirheumatic, antiseptic, antispasmodic, digestive stimulant, diuretic

The leaves and fruit are rich in volatile oils beneficial for the digestive system, what herbalists call a carminative, useful for bloating, gas, and indigestion. If coriander is added to the diet, these symptoms may reduce. Try a cup of **Coriander Leaf Tea** or **Coriander Seed Tea** half an hour before a meal.

Coriander is a natural treatment for high cholesterol levels. The acids (linoleic, oleic, palmitic, stearic, and ascorbic) found in coriander help to lower "bad" cholesterol (LDL) and raise "good" cholesterol (HDL).[73] Add some coriander to the diet and add the fresh leaves to fruits and vegetables in your juicer.

---

73 P. Dhanapakiam, J. Mini Joseph, V. K. Ramaswamy, M. Moorthi, and A. Senthil Kumar, "The Cholesterol Lowering Property of Coriander Seeds (*Coriandrum sativum*): Mechanism of Action," *Journal of Environmental Biology, Journal of Environmental Biology* (January 2008).

Regular consumption of coriander has been shown to reduce blood pressure in many patients suffering from hypertension.[74]

The volatile oils in coriander possess antirheumatic and anti-arthritic properties.

Cineole, a phytochemical found in coriander, is thought to have an anti-inflammatory effect. For arthritis and rheumatism, use some coriander in the diet, apply a coriander salve (see page 16) or **Coriander Infused Oil** topically to the affected areas, or pulverise the leaves and use as a poultice.

The volatile oils found in fresh coriander leaves are antiseptic, antimicrobial, and healing, and a rinse of double-strength **Coriander Leaf Tea** will help treat mouth ulcers.

A well-known home remedy for conjunctivitis is to bathe the closed eyelids with **Coriander Seed Tea**.

CAUTION: Coriander is considered safe in food amounts and when taken by mouth in appropriate medicinal amounts for most people. When coriander comes in contact with the skin, it can cause skin irritation and inflammation or an allergic reaction in some people. As always, if you are pregnant or breastfeeding, stay on the safe side and stick to food amounts. Coriander can marginally lower blood sugar levels, so if you are diabetic, you should monitor these carefully. It can also slightly lower blood pressure, so if you take medications for hypertension or have low blood pressure, monitor your levels carefully.

---

74   Qaiser Jabeen, Samra Bashir, Badiaa Lyoussi, and Anwar H. Gilani, "Coriander Fruit Exhibits Gut Modulatory, Blood Pressure Lowering and Diuretic Activities," *Journal of Ethnopharmacology* 122, no. 1 (25 February 2009): 123–130.

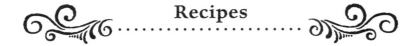

Recipes

Coriander Leaf Tea

1 TABLESPOON FRESH CORIANDER (CILANTRO) LEAVES

250 MILLILITRES (1 CUP) BOILING WATER

Pour the boiling water over the leaves. Cover and infuse for five minutes, strain, and drink.

Coriander Seed Tea

1 TEASPOON CORIANDER SEEDS

250 MILLILITRES (1 CUP) WATER

Lightly crush the seeds and put in a pan with the water. Simmer for fifteen minutes, remove from the heat, and leave to stand for another five to ten minutes. Strain and drink.

Hippocras

1 LITRE (4 CUPS) RED WINE

5 TABLESPOONS SUGAR

½ TEASPOON GINGER

½ TEASPOON POWDERED CINNAMON

⅛ TEASPOON CLOVES

1 TEASPOON GROUND CORIANDER SEEDS

Slightly warm the wine but do not boil or all the alcohol will disappear. Add the sugar and spices and stir to dissolve. Heat very gently for ten to fifteen minutes. Serve warm or cold.

. . . .
Coriander Infused Oil

1 TABLESPOON CORIANDER SEEDS, CRUSHED

250 MILLILITRES (1 CUP) VEGETABLE OIL

In a double boiler, put in the seeds and cover with vegetable oil. Simmer very gently, covered, for two hours. Turn off the heat and allow the oil to cool before straining. If you wish, you can add fresh herbs to the oil. Repeat the process for a stronger oil.

. . . .
Love Incense

½ PART CORIANDER SEEDS, CRUSHED

½ PART CARDAMOM PODS, CRUSHED

¼ PART CINNAMON STICKS, CRUSHED

¼ PART GINGER POWDER

½ PART DRIED LEMON PEEL, CHOPPED

3 PARTS FRANKINCENSE (OPTIONAL)

Blend together and burn on charcoal.

. . . .
Coriander Flower Essence

Gather mature coriander flowers. Float them on the surface of 150 millilitres spring water in a bowl and leave in the sun for three or four hours. Make sure that they are not shadowed in any way. Remove the flowers. Pour the water into a bottle and top up with 150 millilitres brandy or vodka to preserve it. This is your mother essence. To make up the flower essences for use, put seven drops from this into a 10-millilitre dropper bottle, and top that up with brandy or vodka. The usual dose is four drops of this in a glass of water four times a day. When making this it is important not to handle the flowers. It is the vibrational imprint of the flowers you want to be held by the water, not your own imprint.

. . . . .

Cumin

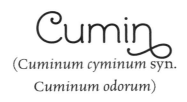

(Cuminum cyminum syn. *Cuminum odorum)*

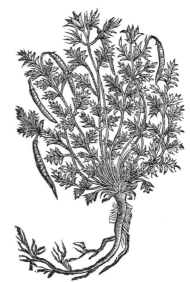

PLANETARY RULER: Mars

ELEMENT: Fire

ASSOCIATED DEITIES: None

MAGICAL VIRTUES: Love, faithfulness, fidelity

Originally cultivated in Iran and the Mediterranean region, cumin is often confused with caraway (*Carum carvi*), and many European languages do not differentiate between the two. It is frequently impossible to know whether cumin or caraway is referred to in older books, recipes, and folklore. Cumin is mentioned several times in the Bible, though it is sometimes mistranslated as caraway, which was unknown in the region at the time. Then again, the completely unrelated *Nigella sativa* seeds are sometimes called black cumin. Indeed, the seeds of caraway and cumin are quite hard to tell apart, though cumin seeds are larger, oval-shaped, and light brown in colour, with a stronger aromatic flavour than caraway.

The magical virtues of cumin are often conflated with those of caraway seeds. Like caraway, cumin is said to be detested and feared by the fairy folk of Germany, though it is likely that the association originally applied to caraway.

The Greek philosopher Socrates considered cumin beneficial as an aid to scholarly pursuits, while Pliny wrote that the smoked seeds could cultivate a scholarly pallor that just implied long hours of scholarly pursuits, and his students used it to try to make him believe that they were overworked.[75]

The primary magical virtues of cumin are faithfulness and fidelity. In Egypt cumin seeds were sometimes carried in pockets by soldiers and merchants to remind them of those waiting for them back home.[76] In mediaeval Europe it was said that cumin seeds prevented lovers from straying. To ensure their men returned home, young women gave their sweethearts bread seasoned with cumin or wine with cumin, and cumin was baked into the loaves of bread sent with soldiers off to war. It often featured at weddings and was believed that a happy life awaited the bride and groom who carried cumin seeds throughout the wedding ceremony. At Hindu weddings today, cumin seeds and brown sugar are crushed together into a paste and placed in a betel leaf; as the priest recites Vedic mantras, the bride and groom in turn place the leaf on the other's head. The mixture represents the bitterness and sweetness of life. This ceremony should also remind the couple that their relationship is unbreakable and inseparable. Cumin seeds can be baked into cakes and breads to keep a lover faithful or added to handfasting and wedding food and wine. Alternatively, just pop a few seeds in your lover's pocket.

CULINARY USES

Pliny listed cumin as "the best appetizer of all condiments"[77] and in Greece and Rome, a dish of cumin seeds was placed on the table to be used much as pepper is today.

Cumin is used as a flavouring agent in cheeses, pickles, sausages, soups, stews, curries, chilli powders, stuffings, rice and bean dishes, biscuits, cakes, and liqueurs. Grind the seeds just before use and use sparingly, as the taste is strong.

COSMETIC USES

Cumin is wonderful for the skin, a rich source of vitamin E, which helps the skin repair itself and fight the free radical damage that causes wrinkles, sagging, and age spots. Use a teaspoon of freshly ground seeds mixed with a tablespoon of honey as a naturally antibacterial and lightly exfoliating facial scrub. Dab **Cumin Vinegar** on spots and boils.

---

75 Grieve, A Modern Herbal.
76 Spices of Life in Ancient Egypt, http://www.history.com/news/hungry-history/spices-of-life
    -in-ancient-egypt, accessed 26 September 17.
77 Pliny the Elder, The Natural History.

MEDICINAL USES

ACTIONS: anodyne, antacid, anticonvulsant, antidiabetic, anti-inflammatory, antimicrobial, antioxidant, antispasmodic, astringent, bronchodilator, carminative, digestive stimulant, diuretic, emmenagogue, expectorant, galactogogue, sialagogue

The antispasmodic activity of cumin helps with minor digestive problems. The aroma, which comes from an organic compound called cuminaldehyde, activates the salivary glands, while its thymol stimulates bile secretion, so it improves digestion. Add to food or take a cup of **Cumin Tea** half an hour before eating.

Cumin acts as an expectorant, meaning that it loosens up the accumulated phlegm and mucus in the respiratory tracts, making it useful for coughs and colds. It is also a rich source of vitamin C and iron, both of which can help recovery, while the volatile oils present are antiviral. Take a spoonful of **Cumin Electuary** as required, or drink some **Cumin Tea**.

CAUTION: Cumin is a culinary herb and is generally considered safe in food amounts and nontoxic in moderate doses. Allergic reactions to the herb can occur in people who are allergic to other plants in the Apiaceae family. To be on the safe side, it should not be used in medicinal doses during pregnancy or breastfeeding. It should be avoided by those suffering from oestrogen receptor–positive tumours.

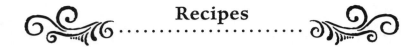

Recipes

Cumin Tea

1 TEASPOON CUMIN SEEDS

250 MILLILITRES (1 CUP) WATER

Lightly grind the seeds and put them in a pan with the water. Bring to boil, then turn off the heat and leave to infuse for fifteen minutes. Strain and drink.

Cumin Vinegar

1 TABLESPOON FRESHLY CRUSHED CUMIN SEEDS

500 MILLILITRES (2 CUPS) CIDER VINEGAR

Combine in a glass jar and leave on a sunny windowsill for three weeks, then strain into a sterilised bottle.

Cumin Electuary

3 TEASPOONS CUMIN SEEDS

1 450-GRAM JAR HONEY

Finely powder the cumin seeds and stir into the honey. Take a teaspoonful one to four times a day.

KEEPING POWDER

3 TEASPOONS CARAWAY SEEDS

3 TEASPOONS CUMIN SEEDS

Finely powder the seeds in a pestle and mortar while keeping your intent in mind. Sprinkle a little of this powder over things you wish to keep safe from being stolen, such as your car, bag, and so on.

SPICY LOVE CHARM BAG

1 TEASPOON CUMIN

½ TEASPOON GINGER POWDER

PIECE DRIED LEMON PEEL

PIECE DRIED ORANGE PEEL

½ TEASPOON POPPY SEEDS

1 VANILLA POD

Sew the ingredients into a pink or red bag, and place under the bed or carry with you to improve your love life.

Dill

Anethum graveolens syn.
Peucedanum graveolens

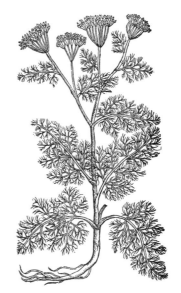

PLANETARY RULER: Mercury

ELEMENT: Air/Fire

ASSOCIATED DEITIES: Mercury, Hermes

MAGICAL VIRTUES: Protection, communication,
mental activity, study, love

The name *dill* comes from the Old Germanic word *dilla*, meaning "to soothe," which may be an allusion to the herb's well-known soothing effect[78] on the digestive system but also refers to the belief that it is soothing and calming in other ways; ancient Greeks even covered their heads in dill leaves to help them sleep. In folk magic it brings peace in the home. You can hang up a **Dill Peace Talisman** to ensure harmony. If there has been an argument, burn some dill seeds on charcoal to cleanse the atmosphere. Dill was thought to be so powerful in this respect that brides in Flanders wore sprigs of dill on their wedding dresses to ensure a harmonious marriage.

When it comes to romance, dill has a mixed reputation. Hildegard von Bingen praised dill for its ability to suppress sexual impulses, and while Dioscorides thought it was good for many ills, he thought too much caused impotence. Pliny, on the other hand, recommended wild asparagus water mixed with dill as an aphrodisiac. It seems to be a question of quantity—a little promotes lust (particularly if combined with a phallic-looking herb

---

78   D'Andréa, *Ancient Herbs in the J. Paul Getty Museum Gardens.*

like asparagus), while too much is lulling; in this I suppose it can be said to be like alcohol. To promote love and affection, try drinking a little **Dill Love Cup** together—but drink too much and performance might be a problem! You can add three or five dill seeds to a talisman or charm bag for a love spell, combined with other herbs of love if you wish (see appendix 1), or anoint a pink or red candle with **Dill Weed Infused Oil** and burn over three nights. This is a recipe for a loving relationship, rather than for the satisfaction of transitory lust.

Dioscorides called dill the seed of Mercury, the god of communication and messenger of the gods, the trickster, the patron of inventors and intellectual endeavour, as well as the god who transports souls to the otherworld. Culpeper assigned it to the planet Mercury, which rules the mind, intellect, and communication, saying, "Mercury has the dominion of this plant, and therefore to be sure it strengthens the brain."[79] Dill can be used in all rituals and spells designed to aid communication and study, mental clarity, magical writings and travel, including shamanic and trance journeys to other realms, since Mercury is a god of mystery and magic who is a guide on these journeys. The power of dill helps ground ideas and mental energy into the world. Used in an incense with other Mercury herbs (see appendix 1) or drunk as **Dill Seed Tea**, it helps clear the mind and strengthen your personal focus. **Dill Flower Essence** can help when you are trying to make sense of the overload of information that comes with the modern world, assimilating and absorbing it into the bigger picture, connecting to the greater consciousness.

Dill was thought to heal wounds more quickly. Roman gladiators rubbed dill oil into their skin to speed up healing. The Romans believed that dill had fortifying qualities and they covered the food given to gladiators with the herb. In the Middle Ages, injured knights were said to have placed burned dill seeds on their open wounds to speed healing. Use **Dill Seed Tea** when you are in need of strength and healing.

Dill is also a protective herb, used to counter magical attack and negative energy. In the Middle Ages it was used in charms against witchcraft; as Drayton wrote in *Nymphidia*, "Therewith her Vervain and her Dill/That hindereth Witches of their Will."[80] It was one of the Saint John's Eve herbs valued as a protection at the summer solstice, a dangerous time when spirits, fairies, and witches were abroad causing mischief. It can be added to incense used for protection and cleansing sacred space. For modern witches, dill is a sacred herb of Midsummer and can be used in incense, cast on the bonfire, or used in the ritual

---

79   *Culpeper's Complete Herbal.*
80   Michael Drayton, *Nymphidia: Or the Court of Faery* (George Routledge and Sons, 1906).

cup. The seed heads hung in the home bring protection to those who live there. They can be hung in a baby's cradle to protect the child. **Dill Weed Tea** can be used as a wash to cleanse sacred space or added to the ritual cleansing bath. **Dill Protection Potion** can be used to seal protective talismans or wiped around doorways and windows against negative influences.

CULINARY USES

Dill is an aromatic herb with delicate, feathery green leaves. It produces flat brown seeds that have a flavour similar to caraway. Both have been used in cookery since ancient times. The herb is native to the Mediterranean and Black Sea regions, and was introduced into Britain by the Romans. Theophrastus wrote of it as a typical Greek kitchen garden plant along with beets, lettuces, and onions.

In the United States the leaves are referred to as "dill weed," and these are best used fresh, as dried leaves rapidly lose their flavour. They go well with tomato dishes, soups, and sauces. Fresh sprigs are frequently used to garnish Scandinavian open sandwiches and go well in potato salad and coleslaw. The seeds, whole or ground, are used to flavour stews, sauces, breads, cakes, pastries, and pickles, especially German-style pickled cucumbers.

COSMETIC USES

The ancient Egyptians used dill widely in the production of cosmetics and perfumes, while in ancient Greece a dill perfume was a sign of wealth. Dill oil is still used in cosmetics and perfumes, and as a fragrance for detergents and soaps.

Dill seed is one of the few substances that is able to stimulate the production of elastin in the skin, which naturally decreases as we age, leading to sagging.[81] Try using **Dill Weed Infused Oil** as an anti-aging night serum or pound two teaspoons of dill seeds into a powder and mix with a tablespoon of slightly warmed honey. Leave this overnight, then apply to the face and neck (or hands) and leave it on for twenty minutes before rinsing with warm water. Follow with a splash of cold water and moisturise as usual. To treat your body, pour two cups of **Dill Seed Tea** into your bathwater.

To strengthen your nails and improve the appearance of the skin of your hands, soak your hands in double-strength **Dill Seed Tea** for five to ten minutes, rinse, and follow with your usual hand cream.

---

81 V. Cenizo et al., "LOXL as a Target to Increase the Elastin Content in Adult Skin: A Dill Extract Induces the LOXL Gene Expression," https://www.ncbi.nlm.nih.gov/pubmed/16842595, accessed 2 January 18.

MEDICINAL USES

ACTIONS: anti-congestive, antidiabetic, antihistimic, anti-inflammatory, antimicrobial, antioxidant, appetiser, aromatic, carminative, disinfectant, emmenagogue, germicide, hypnotic, sedative, stomachic

As already mentioned, the English word *dill* is related to the Old Germanic word *dilla*, meaning "to lull" or "soothe" because it soothes the stomach. Dill was mentioned in the Ebers Papyrus, an Egyptian herbal dating to c. 1550 BCE, where it was described as a remedy for flatulence, dyspepsia, and constipation. The Romans chewed dill seeds to promote digestion, while the Frankish emperor Charlemagne (742–814 CE) insisted that crystal vials of dill oil be placed on the banquet tables to stop the hiccupping of overindulgent guests. The English herbalist Culpeper commented in his herbal that dill "stays the hiccough...(it) is used in medicines that serve to expel wind, and the pains proceeding therefrom." Commercially available dill water was used for centuries to soothe colic in babies, while adults might have preferred to take dill wine to soothe their upset tummies. Drinking **Dill Seed Tea** or simply chewing dill seeds serves to aid digestion and prevent flatulence. Chewing the seeds stimulates saliva, which is the start of the digestive process, while the carvone present in them freshens the breath owing to its antimicrobial nature.

To discourage urinary tract infections, add some double-strength **Dill Seed Tea** to your bath. A cup of **Dill Seed Tea** can be taken before bed to prevent insomnia and promote restful sleep. The flavonoids and vitamin-B complex in dill are believed to activate the secretion of certain enzymes and hormones which have a calming effect, and this can also be useful for tension headaches.

CAUTION: Dill is considered safe for most people when consumed as a food or taken by mouth as a medicine. However, as dill is used in herbal medicine to start menstruation, it is not safe to take in more than small amounts during pregnancy, and to be on the safe side it should be avoided when breastfeeding. Dill lowers blood sugar marginally, so if you are diabetic, you should monitor your levels carefully. Stop taking medicinal amounts of dill for at least three weeks before surgery. Do not take dill if you are on lithium because it acts as a diuretic and may affect how much lithium is in your body. Fresh dill can cause contact dermatitis in some sensitive people, so exercise care. Fresh dill on the skin can also increase the photosensitivity of the skin, making you sunburn more easily.

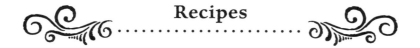

Recipes

DILL SEED TEA

1 TEASPOON CRUSHED SEEDS

250 MILLILITRES (1 CUP) WATER

Put the seeds and water in a pan and simmer for ten minutes. Remove from the heat, leave to stand for five minutes, strain, and drink.

DILL WEED TEA

Add a sprig of dill herb to a cup of boiling water and infuse for ten minutes. The resulting infusion may be added to water for cleansing the sacred space or to the ritual cleansing bath.

DILL WEED INFUSED OIL

Pack a clean glass jar with dill herb. Fill the jar with vegetable oil (such as sunflower) and leave on a sunny windowsill for two weeks. Strain the oil into a clean jar. Stopper tightly and label. Dill oil can be used to seal protective talismans, doorways, and windows against negative influences.

. . . .

DILL PROTECTION POTION

500 MILLILITRES (2 CUPS) BOILING WATER

½ TEASPOON DILL SEEDS, CRUSHED

½ TEASPOON ROSEMARY, CHOPPED

½ TEASPOON BASIL

½ TEASPOON CLOVES, CRUSHED

½ TEASPOON CORIANDER SEEDS, CRUSHED

½ TEASPOON THYME

At the full moon, pour the boiling water over the herbs and seeds and infuse, covered, for twenty minutes. Strain and use to wipe around the doors and windows of your house or any other areas you feel need protecting.

. . . .

DILL LOVE CUP

250 MILLILITRES (1 CUP) RED WINE

1 TEASPOON DILL SEEDS

Put the wine in a saucepan and add the dill seeds. Warm the wine gently for five minutes, but do not boil or all the alcohol will evaporate. Strain and pour into a goblet and share with the one you love. Dill seeds infused in wine are considered to be an aphrodisiac, and magicians traditionally used dill in their love spells. This drink also makes a good loving cup for the couple at a handfasting.

. . . . .

DILL FLOWER ESSENCE

Gather five or six mature flowers. Float them on the surface of 150 millilitres spring water in a bowl and leave in the sun for three to four hours. Make sure that they are not shadowed in any way. Remove the flowers. Pour the water into a bottle and top up with 150 millilitres brandy or vodka to preserve it. This is your mother essence. To make up the flower essences for use, put seven drops from this into a ten-millilitre dropper bottle, and top that up with brandy or vodka. This is your dosage bottle. The usual dose is four drops of this in a glass of water four times a day. When making this, it is important not to handle the flowers—it is the vibrational imprint of the flowers you want to be held by the water, not your own imprint.

DILL PEACE TALISMAN

WHITE BAG

3 TEASPOONS DILL SEEDS

½ TEASPOON CORIANDER SEEDS

3 BASIL LEAVES, DRIED

1 DOVE FEATHER

1 PIECE ROSE QUARTZ

SILVER CORD

On a Sunday, assemble the ingredients and place into the bag, concentrating on the intent of peace and harmony. Tie up the bag with a silver cord. To consecrate, light a charcoal block and set some dill seeds on it to burn, and consecrate the talisman in the smoke.

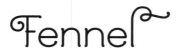Fennel

Foeniculum vulgare syn.
Anethum foeniculum

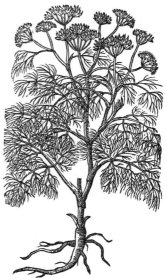

PLANETARY RULER: Mercury

ELEMENT: Fire

ASSOCIATED DEITIES: Apollo, Dionysus, Prometheus, Adonis

MAGICAL VIRTUES: Protection, purification, fertility, shamanic travel, courage, joy

According to Greek mythology,[82] the earliest humans lived naked, cold, and hungry, without hope or inspiration. The Titan Prometheus ("Foresight") felt pity for them and implored the Olympian gods to help, but they refused, saying that they didn't want humans to become more like gods. Deciding to act alone, Prometheus stole fire from the hearth of the gods and, concealing it in a fennel stalk, took it down to the earth. He taught humans how to warm their homes and how to use fire to cook. Bleakness and darkness were now illuminated by light and hope. People learned how to grow food, domesticate animals, craft metal, create art and writing, and pursue philosophy, mathematics, and astronomy. One spark of celestial fire concealed in a fennel stalk made all the difference.

---

82   Hesiod, *Theogony*, online at http://www.perseus.tufts.edu/hopper/text?doc
      =Perseus%3Atext%3A1999.01.0130%3Acard%3D1, accessed 14 December 2017.

Everything is illuminated and vitalised from within a divine spark from the gods; it animates all life. Inspiration sent by the gods is called the "fire in the head," where thought and spirit meet to create something new. Sometimes we feel that the fire within has gone out, and this is when you can utilise the magic of fennel. The abbess Hildegard von Bingen said, "However fennel is eaten, it makes men merry, and gives them a pleasant warmth."[83] If you are feeling stuck, low, and uninspired, **Fennel Seed Tea** can be employed in spells, rituals, and spiritual work to ignite the fire within, or use the seeds and dried herb in spells, rituals, incenses, charm bags, sachets, and talismans. Use **Fennel Flower Essence** if you feel worn down, apathetic, and indecisive; one spark is all that is needed to change a life—or, indeed, the world.

A stalk of giant fennel (*Ferula communis*) capped with a pine cone formed the thyrsus,[84] the wand able to "open up channels of life sustaining fluid from the earth"[85] carried by Dionysus, the wild god of fertility, winemaking, the theatre, and the divinely inspired madness that brings about insight and creativity. As the fennel stalk pushes its way from the earth in spring, it is suggestive of an erect phallus, and the thyrsus was a wand used in ritual and dance, a symbol of fertility, prosperity, and pleasure, the pine cone representing the "seed" issuing forth. Sometimes the thyrsus was displayed in conjunction with a wine cup, suggesting a male and female combination. Fennel may be used in spells and rituals of fertility, creative endeavour, vision quests, and shamanic travel. Use **Fennel Metheglin**, **Fennel Seed Tea**, an incense with fennel, put fennel seeds in charm bags and talismans, or use the incense to consecrate talismans. A giant fennel (*Ferula communis*) wand embodies creative energy directly from the gods and may be used to direct energy accordingly.

In Greece fennel also played a part in the Adonia, celebrating another vegetation god, the youthful Adonis, lover of Aphrodite.[86] This took place when, as Theophrastus said, "the sun is at its most powerful" during the dog days of late July.[87] During the festival women would plant small gardens, called Gardens of Adonis, in clay pots or wicker baskets. These were composed of wheat, barley, fennel, and lettuces. The women would climb ladders up to their rooftops, thereby placing the little gardens as close to the sun as they could. At this time of year the great heat gives an impetus to a plant's growth, but they can become leggy

83   von Bingen, *Causae et Curae*.
84   Rätsch and Müller-Ebeling, *The Encyclopedia of Aphrodisiacs*, and Farrar, *Gardens and Gardeners of the Ancient World*.
85   Segal, *Dionysiac Poetics and Euripides' Bacchae*.
86   Marcel Detienne, *The Gardens of Adonis* (Princeton University Press, 1977).
87   Anna Franklin, *Lughnasa, History, Lore and Celebration* (Lear Books, Earl Shilton, 2010).

· · · · ·

and spindly, with the plant outgrowing its strength while young shoots wither in dryness. When the plants died, the pots were thrown in the river with images of Adonis. These rites were intended to invoke abundant rainfall in the coming season.[88] The gardens were left to grow for only eight days to come to maturity, in contrast to the eight months taken by the cereal crop under the auspices of the grain goddess Demeter. Thereafter August was sacred to the goddess Demeter and her daughter Persephone.[89]

Fennel grows widely in the Mediterranean region, where it was often used as a fodder crop.[90] Both the scientific and Latin names derive from the Latin for "little hay."[91] The town of Marathon, site of the famous battle between the Athenians and the Persians, means "place of fennel." After the battle, the Athenians used woven fennel stalks as a symbol of victory. Roman soldiers mixed fennel seed with their meals to assure fighting strength and courage.[92] Taking **Fennel Seed Tea** or inhaling the fragrance of the seeds is refreshing and revitalising. **Fennel Seed Tea** can be taken when courage and stamina is needed, such as before an initiation or during the Lughnasa games. Wreaths woven from fennel can be used to crown the victorious contestants.

Fennel is a protective herb, used to dispel negative influences. It is one of the sacred herbs mentioned in the Anglo-Saxon Nine Herbs Charm recorded in tenth century CE[93] to treat the "flying venom" thought to cause disease or those who had been "elf shot," or bewitched with illness after being shot with fairy arrows. The nine herbs (fennel, mugwort, cockspur grass [or perhaps betony], lamb's cress, plantain, mayweed, nettle, crab apple, and thyme) were used as a herbal salve with a recited charm, the *Lacnunga*, or Lay of the Nine Herbs. During the Middle Ages fennel was hung over the door on the dangerous Mid-summer's Eve to keep away evil spirits, fairies, and witches. The seeds were also pushed into keyholes in the belief that this would prevent ghosts from entering. For protection and purification, fennel can be used in incenses; add fennel seeds to charms, amulets, and talismans. Add **Fennel Seed Tea** or **Fennel Leaf Tea** to the ritual bath. Use to consecrate amulets or in a wash to cleanse ritual space and magical tools. Use **Fennel Seed Tea** or

88   D'Andréa, *Ancient Herbs in the J. Paul Getty Museum Gardens.*
89   Anna Franklin, *Lughnasa, History, Lore and Celebration* (Lear Books, Earl Shilton, 2010).
90   Michael Stewart, "People, Places and Things: Fennel," Greek Mythology: From the Iliad to the Fall of the Last Tyrant, http://messagenetcommresearch.com/myths/ppt/Fennel_1.html, accessed 25 September 17.
91   Brunton-Seal and Seal, *Kitchen Medicine.*
92   D'Andréa, *Ancient Herbs in the J. Paul Getty Museum Gardens.*
93   Edward Pettit, *Anglo-Saxon Remedies, Charms, and Prayers from British Library MS Harley 585: The "Lacnunga,"* 2 vols. (Lewiston and Lampeter: Edwin Mellen Press, 2001).

fennel infused oil (see page 17) to magically seal doorways and windows and prevent evil from entering.

During fasting, **Fennel Seed Tea** can be drunk to alleviate hunger pangs and ease the shock on the body's digestive system.

CULINARY USES

The ancient Egyptians, Greeks, and Romans all ate fennel's seeds, aromatic leaves, and tender shoots.[94] The shoots were cooked as vegetables, the raw stalks were chopped into salads, and seeds were placed under loaves of bread as they were baked to add flavour.[95]

The seeds, bulb, and leaves are used in cooking. The flowers and feathery leaves can be sprinkled into salads, soups, and sauces. The stems, which resemble celery, have a pleasant anise-like flavour. They can be diced into soups and salads, used for savouring stews and stir-fry vegetables, or eaten like celery sticks. Fennel seeds are used to flavour bread, cakes, pastries, soups, stews, sweet pickles, apple pie, and tomato-based sauces. The fennel "root" you can buy is Florence fennel (*Foeniculum vulgare* var. *dulce*). The edible white bulb is actually stacked leaves and not a root at all.

COSMETIC USES

Fennel has skin-softening and anti-aging properties. Use **Fennel Seed Tea** as a wash to cleanse and tone the skin and to remove grime, excess grease, and dead skin cells. It will firm the skin, tighten pores, and reduce wrinkles. Fennel may be added to moisturising creams and lotions. A cream made from fennel seeds is also mildly antiseptic.

If you wake up with swollen and sore eyes, prepare a cup of **Fennel Seed Tea**, soak a cotton ball in it, and place it over your closed eyelids for ten minutes. Rinse with cold water.

Use **Fennel Seed Tea** as a hair rinse to cleanse chemical residues, revitalise hair, strengthen hair follicles, and treat dandruff and scalp problems.

Rub cellulite patches with a paste of ground fennel seeds and a little water or use the paste as an exfoliant.

Use the ground seeds in a facial steam for acne.

---

94   D'Andréa, *Ancient Herbs in the J. Paul Getty Museum Gardens.*
95   Ibid.

MEDICINAL USES

ACTIONS: antacid, antispasmodic, anti-inflammatory, appetiser, aromatic, carminative, circulatory stimulant, diuretic, emmenagogue, expectorant, galactogogue, laxative, oestrogen modulator, rubefacient, vasodilator

Fennel has been used in healing since ancient times. In the third century BCE the Greek Hippocrates used it as a stomach soother for infant colic, Dioscorides recommended it to nursing mothers, and the Roman naturalist Pliny included the plant in twenty-two remedies.[96] The thirteenth-century Physicians of Myddfai declared that "he who sees fennel and gathers it not, is not a man, but a devil,"[97] while the mediaeval abbess and herbalist Hildegard von Bingen thought that fennel forced a person back into the right balance of joyfulness and that its benefits included good digestion and a good body odour.[98] Is it any wonder that the emperor Charlemagne mandated its growth in every garden?[99]

Fennel contains a compound called fenchone, which helps relax the smooth muscle lining the digestive tract, and is therefore an antispasmodic herb used for gas pains, indigestion, and IBS. Many Indian restaurants have a bowl of fennel seeds provided as an aid to digestion.[100] Chew a few fennel seeds or drink **Fennel Seed Tea** twenty or thirty minutes before a meal to prevent cramping and dispel wind in the gut. It also has anti-acidic properties and is extensively used in commercial antacid preparations. A cup of **Fennel Seed Tea** can help ease heartburn. Commission E (the German equivalent of the FDA) endorses fennel for treating digestive upsets.[101]

It is also used for treating cough and catarrh as **Fennel Seed Tea** is a mild expectorant, containing the phytochemicals cineole and anethole, effective in treating inflammation of the mucous membranes of the upper respiratory tract, helping remove mucus and phlegm from the lungs. **Fennel Syrup** is good for coughs, and double-strength **Fennel Seed Tea** may be gargled for sore throats and hoarseness.

Fennel is a diuretic—it increases urination. Its reputation as a weight loss herb may simply relate to its diuretic action, though fennel seeds have the reputation of supressing appetite. The ancient Greeks called fennel *maraino,* which means "to grow thin," believing

---

96 Castleman, *The New Healing Herbs.*
97 Pughe, *The Physicians of Myddfai.*
98 von Bingen, *Causae et Curae.*
99 https://jonbarron.org/herbal-library/foods/fennel, accessed 13 September 17.
100 Castleman, *The New Healing Herbs.*
101 Ibid.

it contributed to weight loss, while Roman ladies took fennel to prevent obesity.[102] Culpeper also wrote that "all parts of the fennel plant are used in drink or broth to make people lean that are too fat."[103] Fennel was used by those fasting on Christian feast days and was widely employed in old and modern slimming formulas.[104] **Fennel Seed Tea** or **Weight Loss Tea** may be useful if you are dieting.

Fennel has a mildly oestrogenic effect, so it is useful for women going through menopause. Drink **Fennel Seed Tea** and use **Fennel Cream** to combat vaginal dryness.

Eye inflammations such as blepharitis and conjunctivitis can be treated with a compress using cold **Fennel Seed Tea** applied over closed eyelids for ten minutes.

Lastly, a cup of **Fennel Seed Tea** may relieve a hangover.

> Caution: Fennel is considered safe for most people, but do not use on
> children and avoid if you have bleeding disorders, hormone-sensitive
> cancers, are taking tamoxifen, and have endometriosis or uterine fibroids.
> Fennel may slightly decrease the effectiveness of birth control pills. Pregnant
> women should not take fennel as a medicinal herb internally as it is a uterine
> stimulant, though small amounts used in cooking are considered safe.

102   Castleman, *The New Healing Herbs*.
103   Culpeper, *Culpeper's Complete Herbal*.
104   Brunton-Seal and Seal, *Kitchen Medicine*.

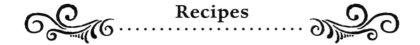

Recipes

FENNEL SEED TEA

1 TEASPOON FENNEL SEEDS, SLIGHTLY CRUSHED

250 MILLILITRES (1 CUP) BOILING WATER

Infuse ten minutes in a covered container, strain, and drink.

FENNEL FACE MASK

3 TABLESPOONS FENNEL SEEDS, CRUSHED

80 MILLILITRES (⅓ CUP) WATER

100 GRAMS (¾ CUP) GROUND OATMEAL

4 TABLESPOONS RUNNY HONEY

Put the fennel seeds in a pan with the water. Bring to boil and remove from the heat. Allow to infuse twenty minutes, then strain off the liquid. Combine this liquid with the oats and honey to make a thick paste. Apply to the cleansed skin of your face and neck. Leave fifteen minutes and then rub gently. Rinse off with warm water.

FENNEL LEAF TEA

2 TEASPOONS FRESH LEAVES

250 MILLILITRES (1 CUP) BOILING WATER

Infuse five minutes, strain, and drink.

. . . .

Weight Loss Tea

1 TEASPOON FENNEL SEEDS, LIGHTLY CRUSHED

1 SPRIG FRESH PARSLEY

1 GREEN TEA BAG OR PINCH OF GREEN TEA

250 MILLILITRES (1 CUP) BOILING WATER

Infuse ten minutes in a covered container, strain, and drink.

. . . .

Fennel Syrup

3 TEASPOONS FENNEL SEEDS

300 MILLILITRES (1¼ CUPS) WATER

250 GRAMS (1 CUP) SUGAR

To make the syrup, first make a fennel decoction by crushing fennel seeds and boiling them in water for ten minutes. Remove from the heat, strain out the seeds through muslin, and measure out 250 millilitres of the decoction (we started with more water to allow for evaporation). Add sugar and heat gently until the sugar is dissolved. Simmer gently until thickened. Pour into sterilised bottles and label. This will keep six to twelve months, unopened, in a cool, dark place. Once opened, keep in the fridge for one to two months. If you wish, you can use honey instead of sugar.

. . . .

Fennel Flower Essence

Gather five mature flowers. Float them on the surface of 150 millilitres spring water in a bowl and leave in the sun for three or four hours. Make sure that they are not shadowed in any way. Remove the flowers. Pour the water into a bottle and top up with 150 millilitres brandy or vodka to preserve it. This is your mother essence. To make up your flower essences for use, put seven drops from this into a ten-millilitre dropper bottle, and top that up with brandy or vodka. This is your dosage bottle. The usual dose is four drops of this in a glass of water four times a day.

. . . . .

FENNEL CREAM

100 MILLILITRES (7 TABLESPOONS) SOLID COCONUT OIL

2 TEASPOONS FENNEL SEEDS, CRUSHED

10 MILLILITRES (2 TEASPOONS) VITAMIN E OIL

In a double boiler, put the coconut oil and crushed fennel seeds. Simmer gently for sixty minutes. Strain through a double layer of muslin into a sterilised jar. When slightly cool but before it sets, stir in the vitamin E oil. This balm helps lubricate the vaginal walls and reduce sensitivity. Fennel has an oestrogenic effect, coconut oil helps restore the body's natural hydration, and vitamin E helps bring back the natural balance.

FENNEL METHEGLIN

3 FENNEL ROOTS

2 SPRAYS RUE

2 KILOS (6 CUPS) HONEY

JUICE OF 2 LEMONS

YEAST AND NUTRIENT

5 LITRES (21 CUPS) WATER

Wash the fennel roots and boil them for forty minutes in one litre of the water. Strain and return the liquor to the pan with the honey and boil for two hours. Skim off any scum and then add the rue. Cool to lukewarm and add the lemon juice, yeast, and nutrient. Strain into sterilised demijohns and fit an airlock. After fermentation has finished (after it has stopped bubbling), syphon off into a clean, sterilised demijohn and fit an airlock. After about a year, you can syphon your fennel metheglin into sterilised bottles.

Fenugreek
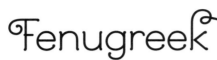

Trigonella foenum-graecum

PLANETARY RULER: Mercury

ELEMENT: Air

ASSOCIATED DEITIES: Apollo, Shitala

MAGICAL VIRTUES: Increase, health, protection, love,
  banishing negativity

The name of this plant comes from *foenum-graecum*, meaning "Greek hay," as the plant was often used as an additive to hay because cattle and horses both love it. The cavalry units of Imperial Rome carried it with them to use as a treatment for sick horses. In Britain fenugreek was employed by the Horseman's Word, or Society of Horsemen, an initiatory secret organisation amongst those who worked with horses during the nineteenth century that used "magical" rituals to control horses. Most of these techniques were based on the horse's sharp sense of smell. Certain substances placed in front of the horse or on the animal itself would cause it to refuse to move forward. This technique is known as jading and is still used by horse trainers today. One stopping oil included cumin seed, celandine, feverfew, fenugreek, and horehound.[105] Fenugreek can be used to work with horse familiars and power animals.

Fenugreek's primary magical power is that of increase—increasing love, increasing prosperity, increasing health, increasing breast milk, and even, reputedly, increasing the

---

105   George Ewart Evans, *Horse Power and Magic* (London: Faber, 1979).

size of a woman's breasts. Use it in spells, rituals, and charms when you want something to increase. Try sprouting some fenugreek seeds as a spell of increase. You can add fenugreek to a **Money-Drawing Incense** or oil, anoint a green candle with **Fenugreek Infused Oil** and burn it, or put it in sachets, charm bags, and talismans to draw prosperity.

In both ancient and modern lore, fenugreek is considered an aphrodisiac, increasing libido in men. You can try adding some fenugreek to food and drink or use in spells and rituals of lust.

While drawing and increasing positivity, fenugreek repels negativity. It was used in the ancient Egyptian town of Esna to repel Apophis, the most dangerous god of chaos and darkness who constantly threatened the divine order. Images of the god were burned with fenugreek and bryonia to banish him.[106] You can use fennel seeds in rituals and spells to drive back chaos and negativity. Try writing down something you wish to be rid of—a bad habit, for example—and burning the paper along with some fenugreek seeds on some charcoal on a fireproof dish. If you feel as though life has slipped off-course and that you have had a run of bad luck because you are not aligned with your cosmic life path, try working with the energy of fenugreek in the form of **Fenugreek Seed Tea**, anointing your forehead with **Fenugreek Infused Oil,** and meditating while burning fenugreek seeds.

In Hindu mythology fenugreek is associated with Shitala Devi ("She Who Cools"), the goddess who cures childhood diseases. In representations of her, she has four hands holding a short broom, a winnowing fan, a jar of cooling water, and a drinking cup. All tin, brass, and clay pots are believed to be filled with the power of the goddess, fertility, and healing. When a ritual pitcher is installed in a temple, it is filled with Ganges water and offerings such as fenugreek and aniseed are presented. Use in spells and rituals of healing.

CULINARY USES

Fresh fenugreek seeds are used as flavouring for curry spice, added to bread, roasted as a coffee substitute, and used to flavour drinks or give a maple flavouring to confectionery. The seeds may be sprouted and the shoots used as salad greens, as they are in Egypt, or cooked.

COSMETIC USES

Julius Caesar mentioned an ointment called *telinum* made from fenugreek and called it soothing. Pliny wrote of it as an ingredient in *myrtinum* (myrtle unguent), among the most popular Egyptian unguents of his time. The ancient world knew the power of fenugreek to

---

106 Ian Rutherford, *Animal Sacrifice in the Ancient Greek World* (Cambridge University Press, 2017).

improve the skin and diminish wrinkles. One Egyptian fenugreek oil was said to transform "an old man into a young man"—at least on the outside.[107]

Fenugreek softens and soothes the skin. It contains lecithin, a natural lipid. Cosmetics manufacturers often add lecithin to products as a skin-conditioning agent and emulsifier. The seeds also have antibacterial and anti-inflammatory properties and are rich in vitamin B3, which helps repair damaged skin cells and regenerate new ones. Grind the seeds and add honey to use as a homemade facial scrub, or use **Fenugreek Infused Oil** as a night serum. You can apply a **Fenugreek Poultice** mixture as a face pack.

The nicotinic acid in fenugreek seeds stimulates hair growth, and the lecithin soothes and shines it. Use **Fenugreek Infused Oil** as a hot oil treatment, or use **Fenugreek Seed Tea** as a hair rinse.

MEDICINAL USES

ACTIONS: anti-inflammatory, anti-pyretic, antispasmodic, demulcent, digestive, emollient, galactogogue, hypoglycaemic, immune stimulant

In Chinese medicine fenugreek is used mainly as a restorative in chronic fatigue and sexual debility. In Islamic medicine the seed is such a treasured tonic that the prophet Mohammed said, "If you knew the value of the fenugreek, you would pay its weight in gold."[108] Dioscorides advocated fenugreek for all types of gynaecological disorders. In the Middle East many nursing mothers take fenugreek seed to increase the flow of milk.

Fenugreek seeds contain a high percentage of mucilage, which is not absorbed by the body but instead passes through the intestines and triggers intestinal muscle contractions. Therefore, fenugreek is a mild but effective laxative. This makes it helpful in treating constipation.

Fenugreek's soothing mucilage helps to relieve a sore throat and hoarseness. Drink or gargle with **Fenugreek Seed Tea** with the addition of a squeeze of lemon juice and a teaspoon of honey.

Fenugreek contains the chemicals diosgenin and oestrogenic isoflavones, which are similar to the female sex hormone, oestrogen. Loss of oestrogen causes menopausal symptoms. Eating fenugreek and drinking **Fenugreek Seed Tea** can be useful for menopausal symptoms.

A **Fenugreek Poultice** may benefit rheumatism and arthritis.

---

107 Lise Manniche, *An Ancient Egyptian Herbal* (University of Texas Press, 1999).
108 https://www.islamicmedicineacademy.co.uk, accessed 10 November 2017.

CAUTION: Fenugreek is considered safe for people when taken by mouth in amounts normally found in food, and for most people in medicinal amounts for a period of up to six months. Side effects can include diarrhoea, stomach upset, bloating, gas, and a "maple syrup" odour in urine. Pregnant women should not take fenugreek by mouth. Large amounts of fenugreek can lower blood sugar, so be careful if you are diabetic or hypoglycaemic. Large amounts of fenugreek should not be taken with antiplatelet or anticoagulant drugs as it may increase the effect of the drugs. Individuals who have allergies to peanuts or soybeans may also be allergic to fenugreek. Repeatedly applying topical fenugreek to the same areas may cause itching, redness, or a rash in some people.

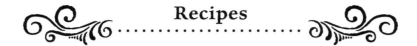

Recipes

FENUGREEK SEED TEA

1 TEASPOON FENUGREEK SEEDS, LIGHTLY GROUND

250 MILLILITRES (1 CUP) COLD WATER

Soak together overnight. Strain the seeds out of the liquid before drinking the tea, which can be warmed or drunk cold.

FENUGREEK INFUSED OIL

2 TABLESPOONS FENUGREEK SEEDS, CRUSHED

500 MILLILITRES (2 CUPS) VEGETABLE OIL

Lightly grind the fenugreek seeds. Put them in a double boiler and cover with the vegetable oil. Simmer very gently, covered, for two hours. Turn off the heat and allow the oil to cool before straining into a sterilised bottle.

FENUGREEK FACE MASK

1 TABLESPOON FENUGREEK SEEDS

2 TABLESPOONS YOGURT (SOY YOGHURT IS FINE)

Grind the fenugreek seeds. Add the yoghurt and let sit for three hours. Apply to your face and neck and leave for thirty minutes. Rinse with warm water and follow with a splash of cold water and a moisturiser.

FENUGREEK POULTICE

50 GRAMS (¼ CUP) FRESHLY GROUND FENUGREEK SEEDS

1 LITRE (4 CUPS) BOILING WATER

Combine and stand until the mixture makes a thick gel. Apply to the desired area and cover with a cotton cloth.

· · · · · · · · · · · · · ·
PROTECTION CHARM BAG

9 FENUGREEK SEEDS

3 LEAVES DRIED BASIL

2 BLACK PEPPERCORNS

1 RED CHILLI (DRIED)

7 CLOVES

5 DILL SEEDS

PIECE OF DRIED LEMON PEEL

Sew into a white bag, holding your intent in your mind as you assemble and create this charm. The bag can be hung up by the door of your house to protect it or carried when you feel you need protection in difficult situations.

· · · · · · · · · · · · · ·
MONEY-DRAWING INCENSE

½ PART FENUGREEK, CRUSHED

¼ PART BASIL, DRIED AND SHREDDED

½ PART CINNAMON STICKS, CRUSHED

⅛ PART CLOVE, CRUSHED

½ PART GINGER POWDER

½ PART ORANGE PEEL, DRIED AND SHREDDED

FEW DROPS ORANGE ESSENTIAL OIL (OPTIONAL)

3 PARTS FRANKINCENSE (OPTIONAL)

Blend together and burn on charcoal.

Garlic

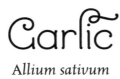

Allium sativum

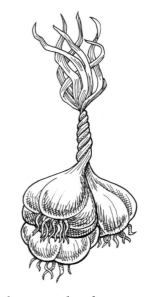

PLANETARY RULER: Mars

ELEMENT: Fire

ASSOCIATED DEITIES: Hecate, Aesculapius, Mars,
Zeus Kasios, Sokar, Osiris, Ptah, chthonic deities

MAGICAL VIRTUES: Apotropaic (able to ward off evil
spirits), protection, healing, strength, courage, aphrodisiac

In Muslim lore, as the Devil left the Garden of Eden, where he stepped garlic sprang from beneath one foot and onion from the other.[109] Similarly, in the Bower Manuscript, a medical treatise of the fifth century CE, garlic is identified as having sprung from the blood of a demon, an enemy of the gods who was killed by Vishnu.[110] In Hindu philosophy onion and garlic are foods with the quality of *tamas* ("darkness") about them. Indeed, there is a common belief that garlic and onions are tied to underworld forces, death, darkness, and evil.

The first thing anyone notices about garlic is the pungent smell. The ancient Greek name for garlic was *scorodon*, and the French physician Henri Leclerc (1870–1955), who coined the term *phytotherapy* for the therapeutic application of herbal medicines, thought

---

109 Grieve, *A Modern Herbal.*

110 A. F. R. Hoernle (ed.), *The Bower Manuscript, Archaeological Survey of India* (Calcutta: New Imperial Series 22, 1893).

this must derive from *skaion rodon*, which he translated as "stinking rose," though this is fanciful.

Whereas sweet perfumes such as frankincense are thought pleasing to the gods in most cultures, more pungent odours are believed to offend them, or even to be polluting to the spirit. Therefore, those coming into the presence of the gods—in a temple, for example—had to be clean and fragrant, and not stink of sweat or garlic and onions.[111] In ancient Greece people who had eaten garlic were not permitted to enter certain temples of Cybele, while in Babylon they were banned from the shrine of the god Nabu.[112] Plutarch wrote that priests refused to eat garlic and onions as they are the only plants that flourish at the dark of the moon, and they are "suitable for neither fasting nor festival because in the one case it causes thirst and in the other tears for those who partake of it."[113] In modern India garlic and onions are considered impure offerings to the Hindu gods. Yogis, orthodox Hindus, and Jains reject garlic as being too stimulating, therefore rooting the consciousness more firmly in the body and interfering with meditation. Chinese Buddhists refrain from eating garlic in the hope that this will reduce sexual desire and contribute to purity.[114] In nineteenth-century China officials participating in state ceremonies were expected to abstain from any foods that made them "impure," which included garlic, leeks, and onions.[115]

Perhaps because of the sulphurous smell, because they grow underground as bulbs, or because they provoke tears akin to mourning, onions and garlic were associated with death and chthonic deities. In Egypt onions were used while embalming people, placed on the eyes and inside the ears to mask the smell.[116] During the festivals of the god Sokar (Seker), the lord of tomb entrances depicted as a mummified hawk, his followers had strings of onions around their necks, referencing his underworld nature. According to Pliny, garlic and onions were invoked as deities by the Egyptians at the taking of oaths.[117]

Garlic was considered a suitable offering for the underworld forces, whether evil spirits, demons, or chthonic deities, to seek their protection, divine their intentions, or to repel them and eliminate the evils they brought. The ancient Greeks offered garlic to the witch

111 Samuel Daiches and Israel W. Slotki (trans.), *Kethuboth: The Babylonian Talmud* (London: Soncino Press, 1936).
112 Simoons, *Plants of Life, Plants of Death*.
113 Plutarch, Isis, and Osiris, online at http://penelope.uchicago.edu/Thayer/E/Roman/Texts/Plutarch/Moralia/Isis_and_Osiris*/home.html, accessed 11 November 17.
114 Simoons, *Plants of Life, Plants of Death*.
115 Stuart E. Thompsom, *Death, Food and Fertility in Death Ritual in Late Imperial and Modern China*, (University of California Press, 1988).
116 Gahlin, *Gods and Myths of Ancient Egypt*.
117 Pliny the Elder, *The Natural History*.

goddess Hecate, who could cause or cure a host of banes. Theophrastus commented that superstitious Greeks placed wreaths of garlic on crossroad altars to the goddess Hecate, and she was believed to punish with madness anyone who dared to eat her suppers.[118] Despite the advent of Christianity, these offerings continued into the eleventh century CE, and there are reports of the church trying to stamp them out. Hecate is often said to have led the witch rides of mediaeval times.[119]

In ancient Greece garlic was considered a powerful force against the evil eye.[120] This continued into modern times, and Greeks might attach a cluster of garlic over the door of the house or shop to protect against the evil eye.[121] Infants and children were thought to be at especial risk, and Greek midwives would take garlic into the delivery room and tie some around the child's neck to protect it[122] while the mother would keep some garlic beneath her pillow.[123] In some parts of Greece, merely uttering the word *garlic* is thought a defence against the evil eye, as is exclaiming "Garlic in your eyes!" after inadvertently saying something unlucky, or directing the phrase at someone suspected of having evil intent.[124] Most Turks wore something to ward off the evil eye, which might be a bead in the shape of an eye or a small sack of garlic and cloves attached to the underclothing with a pin.[125]

Garlic protected against evil and misfortune in other ways. Homer reported that the hero Odysseus owed his escape from the witch Circe to "yellow garlic."[126] It was eaten by ancient Greek and Roman herb collectors before they set out to pluck poisonous herbs such as black hellebore.[127] In ancient Italy it was believed that hen's eggs could be prevented from spoiling during thunderstorms by attaching garlic with iron nails to the chicken pen.[128] This practice was still in use in modern Sicily, where the nail was thought

118   K. F. Smith, "Hecate's Suppers," *Encyclopaedia of Religion and Ethics,* vol. 6 (Edinburgh: T.& T. Clark, 1926).

119   Ibid.

120   R. G. Ussher, *The Characters of Theophrastus* (London: Macmillan, 1960).

121   Margaret M. Hardie, *The Evil Eye: A Folklore Casebook* (NY: Garland, 1981).

122   Ibid.

123   Ibid.

124   Ibid.

125   Rosemary Zumwalt-Levy, "'Let It Go to the Garlic!': Evil Eye and the Fertility of Women among the Sephardim," *Western Folklore* 55, no. 4 (1996).

126   Homer, *The Odyssey.*

127   Dioscorides, *De materia medica,* online at https://archive.org/stream/de-materia-medica/scribd -download.com_dioscorides-de-materia-medica_djvu.txt. Pliny the Elder, *The Natural History.*

128   Columella, "On Agriculture," online at http://www.archive.org/stream/onagriculturewito2coluuoft /onagriculturewito2coluuoft_djvu.txt.

· · · · ·

to absorb noises that might upset the chickens. In modern China people visiting a mortuary wear some garlic about their clothes to protect themselves against the forces of death.

Garlic also protected from the malicious attentions of fairies, demons, and evil spirits. In relatively modern Greece, children born on Christmas Day were thought at risk of becoming one of the *Kallikantzaroi*, evil spirits of chaos that appear during the Twelve Days of Christmas, and to prevent them being taken, the child was wound with braids of garlic.[129] Likewise, at the dangerous time of May Day, when many spirits were about, garlic might be sewn into a child's clothes.[130] In Romania garlic gathered on Trinity Sunday was tied around the neck of a child or tail of an animal to protect them. During Lent, when people were thought most in danger of witches, people smeared garlic on their armpits, the soles of their feet, and breasts at Shrovetide.[131] Seventeenth-century Danish mothers put garlic in their infants' cribs or over the door to protect their children,[132] while Swedish bridegrooms sewed garlic and other strong-smelling herbs in their clothes to protect themselves from trolls and sprites.[133] In Eastern Europe it was common for peasants to hang wreaths of garlic over their doors to protect them from vampires, and in modern India garlic is hung over the door to repel demons.

Garlic was also believed to drive out evil spirits and was used in exorcism. Idols of Chang Ling, the Taoist patriarch of exorcism, represent him with fistfuls of garlic or leeks.[134] In early England a man possessed by a demon was given a potion of garlic, holy water, and church lichen with "Christ's mark or cross," masses were sung over it, and the man took a drink of it from a church bell.[135] In Konkan when a Hindu man is thought possessed by a certain evil spirit, an exorcist squeezes some garlic into the person's ears or up his nostrils.[136]

The disease-fighting properties have been known since ancient times, though its value as an antibiotic, antiviral, and antifungal was not understood. The symbols of the Greek healer-god Aesculapius were the mortar, pestle, garlic, and squill. Before the mechanics of disease and illness were known, they were often thought to be caused by noxious mias-

129 George A. Megas, *Greek Calendar Customs* (Athens: Press and Information Department, 1963).
130 Ibid.
131 Simoons, *Plants of Life, Plants of Death.*
132 Ibid.
133 Ibid.
134 Ibid.
135 Ibid.
136 W. Crooke, *The Popular Religion and Folk-Lore of Northern India*, volume II (London: Archibald Constable and Co., 1896).

mas or the attentions of evil spirits, and it was recognised that garlic combatted them. In Romania the Calusari, a secret society of dancers, dedicated themselves to curing diseases thought to be caused by fairies, such as rheumatism, stroke, plague, and cholera. They worked under the auspices of the fairy queen, Doamna Zinelor, an altered Romanian form of the Roman goddess Diana, whose very name came to mean "fairy" (zina). The Calusari had a flag bearing the image of a bag containing magical herbs, notably garlic and mugwort, most potent against fairies. They chewed as much garlic as they could to protect themselves and spat garlic onto the faces of the afflicted.[137]

Garlic was given to the pyramid builders in ancient Egypt to give them stamina. When they threatened to go on strike, they were given more garlic. In ancient Greece and Rome, garlic was eaten by rural folk as it was believed to provide fortitude and bravery. Virgil observed in his Eclogues that "Thestylus is bruising garlic and wild thyme, strong-smelling herbs for the mowers wearied with the fierce heat."[138] Greek athletes would eat garlic before competing.[139] The belief in the fortifying power of garlic remained a common one; in Paris people used to eat garlic and butter throughout the month of May to strengthen themselves for the coming year.[140] There is an old Welsh saying: "Eat leeks in March and garlic in May, then the rest of the year, your doctor can play."

The Greeks thought soldiers who ate garlic fought better.[141] As Aristophanes said, "Now bolt down these cloves of garlic…Well primed with garlic, you will have greater mettle for the fight!"[142] In Rome garlic was consecrated to Mars, god of war, and it was believed that eating large amounts of garlic made soldiers braver and fiercer. Indeed, the Romans grew garlic in all the lands they conquered.[143] The Greeks also fed garlic to their fighting cocks, as it was thought not only to increase bravery, but also sexual desire, which was considered to increase their aggressiveness.[144]

This brings us on to garlic's reputation as an aphrodisiac. The Roman author Pliny said it gave the body a ruddy colour and should be pounded with fresh coriander and taken in

---

137 Mircea Eliade, "Notes on the Calusari," *The Gaster Festschrift, The Journal of the Ancient Near Eastern Society of Columbia University* 5, 1973.
138 Virgil, *Eclogues*.
139 Simoons, *Plants of Life, Plants of Death*.
140 Ibid.
141 Ibid.
142 Aristophanes, "The Knights," online at https://archive.org/stream/aristophaneswith01arisuoft /aristophaneswith01arisuoft_djvu.txt
143 Simoons, *Plants of Life, Plants of Death*.
144 Ibid.

wine as an aphrodisiac.[145] In one tale by the Greek Aristophanes, some drunken young men went to Megara and kidnapped a prostitute, and the Megarans retaliated by stealing two prostitutes from Aspasia, describing them as being "in agonies of excitement, as though stuffed with garlic."[146] Among practitioners of Ayurvedic medicine today, garlic is held in high regard as an aphrodisiac and for its ability to increase semen.

In modern witchcraft, garlic is used as a herb of protection. Garlic may be hung on the door or in the kitchen to ward off negativity and the evil eye. Cloves of garlic may be placed in protective charms and talismans. Dried and powdered garlic can be added to incense used to drive out negativity or used in exorcism. Garlic is also offered to Hecate and other chthonic deities.

CULINARY USES

A garlic bulb is composed of many individual cloves enclosed in a thin white or purple skin. Garlic has been used as a seasoning for thousands of years and is indispensable in Asian, Indian, and Italian cuisines, among many others, adding a depth of flavour unlike any other. It is usually sautéed with onions and added to soups, stews, casseroles, curries, pasta dishes, vegetable dishes, and so on. For a milder, sweet, nutty taste, garlic can be roasted with the top cut off; wrap the whole bulb in foil and drizzle with olive oil before roasting, then add to pizzas, savoury tarts, spreads, sauces, and hummus. Raw, it imparts a spicy bite and can be added, grated, to dishes just before serving. Use raw in garlic mayonnaise (aioli).

Chew a fresh parsley leaf or a cardamom pod if you are worried about bad breath after eating garlic.

COSMETIC USES

Garlic is antiseptic and astringent, and can be rubbed onto pimples to banish them.

If you can stand the smell, using garlic on your hair and scalp can help prevent hair loss and treat dandruff due to its high levels of allicin, a sulphur compound. Use **Garlic Infused Oil** to massage your scalp on a regular basis. Wash well afterwards!

---

145   Pliny the Elder, *The Natural History*.
146   Athenaeus (Charles Burton Gulick, trans.), *The Deipnosophists* (London: Loeb Classical Library, 1927).

MEDICINAL USES

ACTIONS: anti-atherosclerotic, antimicrobial, antifungal, anti-hypertensive, anti-inflammatory, antioxidant, antiparasitic, antiviral, diaphoretic, diuretic, expectorant, hepato-protective, hypoglycaemic, reduces serum cholesterol, stimulant

Garlic is a broad spectrum antibiotic, killing a wide variety of bacteria. In 1858 Louis Pasteur wrote that garlic was effective even against some bacteria resistant to other factors. Battlefield doctors in both world wars used garlic to disinfect wounds.[147] It is sometimes known as "Russian penicillin" because Russian physicians used it for many years. Dr. Tariq Abdullah stated in the August 1987 issue of *Prevention* that "garlic has the broadest spectrum of any antimicrobial substance that we know of—it is antibacterial, antifungal, antiparasitic, antiprotozoan, and antiviral."[148] Garlic appears to have antibiotic activity whether taken internally or applied topically. It is effective against both gram-positive and gram-negative bacteria, while being harmless to our native gut flora, unlike modern broad-spectrum antibiotics that wipe everything out.[149]

To use garlic as an antibiotic and antiviral, take it internally in the form of **Garlic Vinegar** or **Garlic Electuary**, add some fresh garlic when you juice fruit and vegetables, or just eat a clove of fresh, raw garlic a day, especially if you have a cough or cold or urinary infection.

For external use, apply a garlic poultice on the affected area. Externally, a fresh, peeled, sliced clove of garlic can be applied directly to insect bites, boils, and unbroken chilblains.

Taken regularly, garlic can also help reduce cholesterol and lower blood pressure. It slows arterial plaque formation and clots and may help prevent thrombosis and atherosclerosis. It is a circulatory tonic, increasing blood flow. Garlic exerts a powerful protective action of the heart and also reduces the risk of stroke.

Regular use may help to regulate intestinal flora and combat *Candida albicans*, diarrhoea, stomach cramps, flatulence, and sluggish bowels.

The regular consumption of garlic may be of benefit in reducing the symptoms of rheumatism and arthritis.

147　Rachel Warren Chadd (ed.), 1001 *Home Remedies* (London: Readers Digest, 2005).
148　Quoted in Paul Bergner, "*Allium sativum*: Antibiotic and Immune Properties," *Medical Herbalism: Journal for the Clinical Practitioner*, 1995.
149　Brunton-Seal and Seal, *Kitchen Medicine*.

It has significant antifungal properties, which make it a good treatment for athlete's foot, ringworm, and other fungal skin diseases. Apply **Garlic Infused Oil** directly or use double-strength **Garlic Tea** to make a compress.

Garlic is a popular home remedy for ear infections. Take some **Garlic Infused Oil**, warm a small amount in a spoon, and suck into a dropper. Place two drops in the ear canal and plug with cotton wool. Repeat hourly as needed.

A poultice of fresh crushed garlic applied to warts has powerful antiviral properties, and repeated application can get rid of warts.

CAUTION: Garlic is considered safe for most people, though it can cause bad breath, heartburn, and gas. It should not be applied in high concentrations to the skin as it may cause a burning sensation. To be on the safe side, it should not be taken in medicinal amounts when pregnant or breastfeeding or by young children. Avoid large amounts if you are on blood-thinning medications such as warfarin and for two weeks before surgery. As garlic can lower blood pressure and blood sugar, treat with caution if you are on blood pressure medication or are diabetic. Garlic can decrease the effectiveness of some HIV/AIDS medications and oral contraceptives.

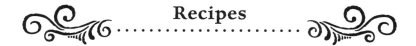

Recipes

Garlic Electuary

1 HEAD OF GARLIC

1 450-GRAM JAR HONEY

Peel and crush the garlic, then add it to the jar of honey. Stir well and seal. This makes a good antibiotic cough "syrup," or it can be applied directly to cuts and scrapes.

Garlic Oxymel for Colds and Flu

1-2 HEADS OF GARLIC

4 CENTIMETRES FRESH GINGER

2 TABLESPOONS FRESH SAGE LEAVES OR 1 TABLESPOON DRIED

250 MILLILITRES (1 CUP) HONEY

1 HEAPED TEASPOON CUMIN SEEDS

250 MILLILITRES (1 CUP) CIDER VINEGAR

Peel the garlic and chop the individual cloves. If you have a large garlic bulb, one will do, or use two small ones. Peel and grate the ginger. Chop the sage leaves. Put the garlic, ginger, and sage into a jar. Pour on the honey. Lightly crush the cumin seeds in pestle and mortar and put these in a pan with the vinegar. Gently warm through without boiling for a few minutes. Pour this into the jar with the rest of the ingredients. Fit a non-metal lid (vinegar will corrode the metal and taint your oxymel) and keep in a cool, dark place for two to three weeks, shaking daily. Strain though muslin into a sterilised jar. Take one or two teaspoons, dissolved in warm water, as needed when you feel the onset of a cold, flu, or sore throat.

GARLIC VINEGAR

FRESH GARLIC

CIDER VINEGAR

Peel and chop your garlic, place in a clean glass jar, and cover completely with the vinegar. Allow this to infuse two weeks in a cool, dark place. Strain into sterilised bottles.

GARLIC INFUSED OIL

GARLIC

OLIVE OIL

Peel and finely chop a bulb of fresh garlic. Put in a pan with enough olive oil to cover. Warm very gently for an hour. Cool. Strain into a sterilised bottle.

GARLIC TEA

2 FRESH GARLIC CLOVES, CRUSHED

250 MILLILITRES (1 CUP) BOILING WATER

Infuse together for five minutes. Strain and drink.

GARLIC ANTIVIRAL TINCTURE

4 CLOVES GARLIC

1 ONION

2 TABLESPOONS GRATED FRESH GINGER ROOT

4 TEASPOONS FRESH CHILLIES

CIDER VINEGAR

Chop the fruits and vegetables and pack into a jar. Cover with cider vinegar and put on a sunny windowsill for two weeks, shaking daily. Strain through a fine cloth into a sterilised jar and label. Make this in advance of the winter and take a teaspoon up to five times a day when you have an infection.

Ginger

Zingiber officinale

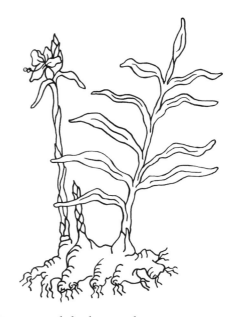

PLANETARY RULER: Mars

ELEMENT: Fire

ASSOCIATED DEITIES: None

MAGICAL VIRTUES: Energy, passion, love,
protection, courage

In the darkest days of winter, with the icy winds whistling around the house, the scent of spicy gingerbread and mulled wine come drifting from the kitchen. Where would Yule be without ginger? It goes in the cake, in the incense, and in the food. Ruled by the element of fire, the magical effect of ginger is to stimulate and speed up action, perfect for restarting the Wheel of the Year, stilled for three days at the solstice. Indeed, ginger energises and accelerates all acts of magic, so add it to spells, rituals, incense, charms, and talismans to make them stronger and swifter in action.

As traditional Chinese medicine has it, ginger restores *yang*, or hot energy. Indeed, the slang meaning of "ginger" implies liveliness and vitality. The "hot energy" it restores has been widely believed to include sexual energy since ancient times, with ginger commonly used as an aphrodisiac. The *Kama Sutra*, a c. 400 BCE Hindu work on human sexuality, suggested ginger as an effective means of exciting sexual energies, while the Greeks and Romans believed it stimulated male sexual arousal. The twelfth-century abbess Hildegard von Bingen, who wrote knowledgeably about herbal remedies, recommended its use for stimulating the vigour of older men married to younger women, while the University of Salerno in Italy taught that to have a happy and vigorous life in old age, including an active sex life, one should eat ginger.[150] All this makes it suitable for tantric rituals and spells of lust, passion, and love. Add powdered ginger to love philtres, incenses, charm bags, and food shared between lovers.

In ancient India ginger was considered both a physical and spiritual cleanser. They shunned bad-smelling onions and garlic before religious ceremonies but ate ginger as its sweet smell made them acceptable to the gods.[151] According to the Koran, ginger is even on the menu in paradise.[152] Eating ginger before ritual is an act of purification, as well as increasing spiritual and magical energy. If you are lucky enough to be able to grow some ginger and have it flower, you can make your own **Ginger Flower Essence** to help you release the wounds of the past and realise your unique value within creation.

Ginger is also a protective herb. In parts of the Malay Peninsula, children wore a piece of ginger around their necks to keep harmful spirits away.[153] At the time of Henry VIII in England, it was believed to ward off plague.[154] Use ginger-infused oil to seal talismans of protection, add ginger root or powdered ginger to protection charms, add powdered ginger to protection incense, and use **Fresh Ginger Tea** as a cleansing ritual wash for tools and magical spaces.

CULINARY USES

Ginger is thought to originate in southeastern Asia, though it is now cultivated commercially in nearly every tropical and subtropical country in the world. It was one of the first spices traded along the spice routes,[155] initially popular for its medicinal qualities and later as a food ingredient. It was certainly known in England before the Norman Conquest (1066 CE), as it was commonly mentioned in eleventh-century Anglo-Saxon medical texts. Like other exotic spices, it was incredibly expensive, with a pound of ginger equivalent to the cost of a sheep in the thirteenth century, but even so, next to black pepper, it was the most popular spice.

We generally know this spice in two forms: dried, powdered ground ginger and the fresh "root" (actually the rhizome of the plant) with its individual divisions, known as

---

150 Swain, *The Lore of Spices*.

151 Castleman, *The New Healing Herbs*.

152 Swain, *The Lore of Spices*.

153 Constance Classen, David Howes, and Anthony Synnott, *Aroma, the Cultural History of Scent* (Routledge, 1994).

154 R. Remadevi, E. Surendran, and P. Ravindran, "Properties and Medicinal Uses of Ginger," in P. Ravindran and K. Babu (eds.), *Ginger: The Genus Zingiber* (Florida, USA: CRC Press, 2005), 489–508.

155 Brunton-Seal and Seal, *Kitchen Medicine*.

"hands." Since they may be imagined as resembling hands with knobbly fingers, this is perhaps why the ancient Greeks and Romans thought it grew in the fabled land of the Troglodytes, a misshapen and promiscuous race living on the edge of the earth.[156] Fresh ginger and ground ginger powder have distinct aromas and properties and are used differently in cooking and in both Ayurveda and traditional Chinese medicine. Ginger root contains a large range of phytochemicals, with the pungency of the fresh root attributed to the primary presence of compounds called gingerols, but when ginger is cooked or dried these turn into shogaols, which are twice as piquant, explaining why dried ginger has a greater pungency than fresh ginger.[157] Cooking also produces zingerone, which is characteristic of the ginger flavour found in gingerbread. Queen Elizabeth I of England is credited with the invention of the gingerbread man, which became a popular Christmas treat.[158] The fresh root is used in both sweet and savoury dishes, but the fiery ground ginger is generally used for baking. Don't be tempted to substitute one for the other in recipes. Fresh ginger is wonderful in stir-fries, curries, sauces, glazes, marinades, ice cream, and all kinds of fruit and vegetable dishes. When buying ginger, look for plump, unwrinkled roots. Store it in the fridge. Replace ground ginger often as it soon loses its piquancy.

If you want to grow ginger at home, you can, but unless you live in a tropical climate it will have to be kept in a warm place indoors. You will often find that the ginger roots you buy from the supermarket will bud and put out a little green shoot. Simply plant this directly into a pot. You can harvest your own ginger rhizomes in about a year.

COSMETIC USES

You may recognise the scent of ginger in commercial cosmetics, particularly men's eau de colognes, but for those of us who like to make our own products, ginger has many benefits. It has antioxidant properties, stimulates circulation to the skin, evens skin tone, and improves skin elasticity, all useful qualities in stopping the appearance of aging. You can use a weekly **Ginger Face Mask**.

If your hair is thinning, ginger may help as it stimulates circulation. Massage your scalp and hair with **Ginger and Cinnamon Massage Oil**.

This quality of stimulating blood flow can help in the battle against cellulite. Use a **Ginger Body Scrub** a couple of times a week.

---

156   Swain, *The Lore of Spices.*
157   http://www.compoundchem.com/2014/11/27/ginger/ accessed 4 October 17.
158   *Herbal Medicine: Biomolecular and Clinical Aspects,* 2nd edition, https://www.ncbi.nlm.nih.gov/books/ NBK92775/ accessed 21 August 17.

MEDICINAL USES

ACTIONS: analgesic, antibacterial, anticoagulant, antiemetic, anti-
inflammatory, antimicrobial, antioxidant, antiparasitic, antispasmodic,
antitussive, anxiolytic, cardiotonic, carminative, circulatory
stimulant, diaphoretic, hypolipidaemic, thermogenic

Ginger has been used medicinally for thousands of years. It featured in the first Chinese great herbal, the Pen Tsao Ching, reportedly compiled by the emperor Shen Nung around 3000 BCE,[159] and is used in half of all traditional Chinese prescriptions.[160] In Ayurveda it is referred to as Mahaousbadba ("great cure") and Visbwa Bhesbaja ("universal medicine"). That tells us just how trusted and useful ginger is.

One of the most common traditional uses is in cases of sickness and diarrhoea. In England from the Middle Ages onwards, **Ginger Beer** was brewed to soothe the stomach, and indeed, it is still used as a home remedy.[161] In fact, doctors and pharmacists will often recommend ginger because it works—it has been shown to be as effective as metoclopramide (an antiemetic drug) in reducing nausea amongst patients receiving chemotherapy.[162] If you are feeling nauseous, sip **Fresh Ginger Tea** throughout the day. It can also be effective in relieving motion sickness—drink some **Fresh Ginger Tea** before you set out on your journey, and chew on a piece of **Crystallised Ginger** while you are travelling.

Ginger's friendliness to the stomach continues with its value as a carminative herb, taken for indigestion, wind, and irritable bowel syndrome. The ancient Greeks took it after large meals, wrapped in sweetened bread to settle the stomach and aid digestion.[163] Add ginger to food and smoothies or drink **Fresh Ginger Tea** after meals.

Ginger is a powerful anti-inflammatory agent, so it is very useful in conditions such as osteoarthritis and rheumatoid arthritis, where inflammation leads to pain. Applied externally, in the form of a compress, salve, or oil, it stimulates peripheral circulation, helping toxins to be removed from painful joints. Furthermore, the topical application of fresh ginger actually has pain-killing properties, with the compound gingerol acting on the receptors located in sensory nerve endings. Applying a **Ginger Compress** to an affected

---

159   Michael Castleman, The New Healing Herbs.
160   Ibid.
161   Castleman, The New Healing Herbs.
162   C. M. Kaefer and J. A. Milner, "Herbs and Spices in Cancer Prevention and Treatment," in I. F. F.
       Benzie and S. Wachtel-Galor (eds), Herbal Medicine: Biomolecular and Clinical Aspects, 2nd edition (Boca
       Raton, FL: CRC Press/Taylor and Francis, 2011), chapter 17.
163   Castleman, The New Healing Herbs.

joint will cause a momentary slight "burn," followed by pain relief.[164] If you are having a flare-up, take a cup of **Fresh Ginger Tea** three times a day and use **Ginger and Cinnamon Massage Oil** or a **Ginger Compress** on affected parts.

A **Ginger Compress** may also help relieve bursitis, tendonitis, and muscle aches and sprains, or rub with **Ginger and Cinnamon Massage Oil**.

Some people find that ginger can help relieve a migraine. Research has found that this is as effective as sumatriptan, a commonly prescribed migraine drug.[165] Ginger is thought to block prostaglandins, the substances that cause inflammation in the blood vessels of the brain.[166] Take a cup of **Fresh Ginger Tea** as soon as you feel any symptoms.

Another traditional use of ginger is to relieve menstrual pain and cramps, and some recent studies bear this out. One showed it was as effective as ibuprofen.[167] Try taking a cup of **Fresh Ginger Tea** as required. It is thought to work by regulating the production of prostaglandins.

In colds, flu, and sinus conditions, ginger loosens phlegm and helps clear mucus from the throat. Drink **Fresh Ginger Tea**, use **Ginger Glycerite**, or have a ginger bath. You can even use a double-strength cup of **Fresh Ginger Tea** as a gargle to relieve a sore throat. The compounds called gingerols in ginger help block the production of the substances that cause bronchial congestion.

> CAUTION: Natural ginger is considered safe for most people, with no known side effects when used moderately or in food amounts. It is best taken with food. However, if you have acid reflux it may exacerbate symptoms. Very large amounts of ginger may marginally lower blood sugar, so if you are diabetic, you should take care to monitor your blood sugar levels. Large amounts of ginger should be avoided by those with gallstones. To be on the safe side, if you wish to use supplemental amounts of ginger during pregnancy, please consult a healthcare professional.

164   M. Zahmatkash et al., "Comparing Analgesic Effects of a Topical Herbal Mixed Medicine with Salicylate in Patients with Knee Osteoarthritis," www.ncbi.nlm.nih.gov/pubmed/22308653, accessed 28 December 17.

165   https://www.ncbi.nlm.nih.gov/pubmed/23657930, accessed 17 December 17.

166   https://migraine.com, accessed 11 October 17.

167   G. Ozgoli, M. Goli, and F. Moattar, "Comparison of Effects of Ginger, Mefenamic Acid, and Ibuprofen on Pain in Women with Primary Dysmenorrhea," https://www.ncbi.nlm.nih.gov/pubmed/19216660, accessed 8 October 17.

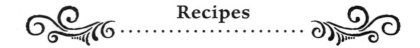

Recipes

Fresh Ginger Tea

2 CENTIMETRES FRESH GINGER

500 MILLILITRES (2 CUPS) WATER

Peel the ginger and slice thinly. Boil the ginger in water for ten to twenty minutes. Remove from heat, strain, and add honey and lemon to taste.

Ginger Compress

Grate 150 grams of fresh ginger and add to a pan of 2 litres water. Simmer gently without boiling for twenty minutes. Strain the ginger water into a heatproof bowl; discard the ginger. Soak a clean cloth in the hot ginger liquid. Wring it out and apply to the affected area. This should be done as hot as is comfortable. When it cools, dip again in the liquid, wring it out, and reapply. You can do this several times. The skin may redden. If you experience itching or discomfort, discontinue use.

Ginger and Cinnamon Massage Oil

1 TABLESPOON FRESH GINGER, PEELED AND CHOPPED

½ TABLESPOON CINNAMON STICKS, CRUSHED

500 MILLILITRES (2 CUPS) VEGETABLE OIL

Place the ginger and cinnamon in a double boiler and cover with the oil. Simmer gently for sixty minutes. Strain your ginger oil into a clean jar.

· · · · · · · · · · ·
GINGER ELECTUARY

Chop fresh peeled ginger. Put in a jar and cover completely with honey. Leave in a warm place for five days. Strain off the honey into a sterilised jar. Discard the ginger. Seal the jar. Take a teaspoon three times a day for coughs and colds.

· · · · · · · · · · ·
ARTHRITIS SMOOTHIE

2 CENTIMETRES FRESH GINGER, PEELED

SMALL PINCH BLACK PEPPER

SMALL PINCH CHILLI POWDER

PINCH CINNAMON POWDER

1 TEASPOON TURMERIC POWDER

2 BANANAS

½ CAN (200 MILLILITRES) COCONUT MILK

100 MILLILITRES (½ CUP) MILK (ALMOND, SOYA, ETC.)

Blend together and drink immediately.

· · · · · · · · · · ·
GINGER GLYCERITE

FRESH ROOT GINGER

VEGETABLE GLYCERINE

Peel and chop the ginger and cover with glycerine. Put on the lid and shake daily. After three weeks, strain into a sterilised bottle. For coughs, colds, sore throats, etc., you can take a spoonful in hot water. Add to sparkling water or soda water and enjoy a ginger mocktail.

. . . .

Ginger Flower Essence

Gather a few mature flowers. Float them on the surface of 150 millilitres spring water in a bowl and leave in the sun for three to four hours. Make sure that they are not shadowed in any way. Remove the flowers. Pour the water into a bottle and top up with 150 millilitres brandy or vodka to preserve it. This is your mother essence. To make up your flower essences for use, put seven drops from this into a 10-millilitre dropper bottle, and top that up with brandy or vodka. This is your dosage bottle. The usual dose is four drops of this in a glass of water four times a day.

. . . .

Crystallised Ginger

50 GRAMS (½ CUP) FRESH GINGER

600 GRAMS (2¾ CUPS) CASTER (SUPERFINE) SUGAR

750 MILLILITRES (3¼ CUPS) WATER

Peel ginger and slice into rounds about half a centimetre thick. Mix the sugar and water in a large pan and bring to boil. When sugar is dissolved, add the ginger and continue to boil for forty-five minutes. Drain the ginger. Carefully put the ginger on a cooling rack and leave to drain and cool for about forty minutes. Toss in caster (superfine) sugar and then spread out on greaseproof paper to dry. Store in airtight container.

You can reserve the liquid as a ginger syrup to take for coughs and colds, or pour it over desserts, ice cream, etc.; mix with soda water and drink; or use to make a cocktail called a Dark and Stormy, mixed with soda water and dark rum and served with a twist of lime.

. . . .

GINGER ALE (ALCOHOLIC)

PEEL AND JUICE OF 2 LEMONS

60 GRAMS (⅔ CUP) ROOT GINGER, BRUISED

450 GRAMS (2¼ CUPS) SUGAR

15 GRAMS (5 TEASPOONS) CREAM OF TARTAR

YEAST AND NUTRIENT

4½ LITRES (19 CUPS) WATER

Peel the lemons, removing all the white pith. Place the peel in a brewing bin with the ginger, sugar, and cream of tartar. Boil 1 litre (4 cups) of the water and pour over the sugar and ginger mix, stirring to dissolve. Allow to cool before adding the lemon juice and yeast and the remaining water. Stir well, cover, and keep in a warm place for a week. Siphon off into pint bottles and add ½ teaspoon sugar to each bottle. Seal them tightly and keep in a warm place for 3 days, then remove to a cool place for storage.

. . . .

OLD-FASHIONED GINGER BEER (NON-ALCOHOLIC)

30 GRAMS (⅓ CUP) GINGER ROOT, PEELED AND CHOPPED

500 GRAMS (2½ CUPS) SUGAR

15 GRAMS (5 TEASPOONS) CREAM OF TARTAR

1 LEMON

7 LITRES (29½ CUPS) WATER, BOILING

1 SACHET BREWING YEAST

Bruise the ginger and put into a plastic brewing bin with the sugar and cream of tartar. Add the juice and zest of the lemon. Pour on the boiling water. Stir to dissolve the sugar. When cooled to lukewarm, add the yeast. Put on the lid and leave in a warm place for twelve hours. Skim off the yeast and syphon off the liquid into plastic bottles, leaving about five centimetres at the top because the brew will create carbon dioxide. Fit screw-on lids and leave in a warm, dark room for about three days. You will need to loosen the caps a couple of times a day, without opening the bottles completely, to let off the pressure. This will create a fizzy pop ready to drink in about four days.

. . . . .

. . . .

Ginger Face Mask

½ TEASPOON POWDERED GINGER

2 TEASPOONS HONEY

½ TEASPOON LEMON JUICE

Mix the powdered ginger, honey, and lemon. Apply to the face, leave thirty minutes, and rinse.

. . . .

Ginger Body Scrub

2 TABLESPOONS SALT OR SUGAR

2 TEASPOONS VEGETABLE OIL

2 TEASPOONS GRATED FRESH GINGER

Combine. Use to gently massage into the skin (avoid the face). This will keep for a week in the fridge.

. . . .

Ginger Syrup

100 GRAMS (1 CUP) FRESH GINGER ROOT, PEELED

1 LITRE (4 CUPS) WATER

RIND OF 1 LEMON

SUGAR

LEMON JUICE

Place the ginger, water and lemon rind into a pan and bring to boil, then simmer gently for forty-five minutes. Strain. To every 500 millilitres (2 cups) of liquid, add 500 grams (2½ cups) of sugar and the juice of one lemon. Put in a clean pan and boil ten minutes. Cool and bottle. For coughs and colds, take one tablespoon in hot water.

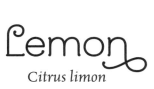
Lemon
Citrus limon

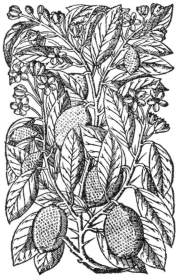

PLANETARY RULER: Moon

ELEMENT: Water

ASSOCIATED DEITIES: Alakshmi

MAGICAL VIRTUES: Protection, dispelling negativity

Despite being associated with the Mediterranean region today, the lemon itself was unknown to the ancient Egyptians, Greeks, and Romans. Citrus fruits originated in southeastern Asia and the Greeks probably first encountered them in the form of citrons during the campaigns of Alexander the Great.[168] The lemon is actually a cultivated hybrid deriving from wild species such as the citron and mandarin, and the first description of the true lemon itself is found in an early tenth-century CE Arabic treatise on farming.[169]

In lore, lemons—and their precursor the citron—have the reputation of dispelling poisons and other negative influences. The Roman Pliny prescribed citron as an antidote to various poisons,[170] and in one tale reported by the writer Athenaeus of two criminals thrown into a pit of snakes, the one that had taken the precaution of eating a citron beforehand survived.[171] The emperor Nero consumed large numbers of citrus fruits as he was

---

168 Margaret Briggs, *Lemons and Limes* (Leicester: Abbeydale Press, 2007).

169 Sarton, *Introduction to the History of Science*.

170 Pliny the Elder, *The Natural History*.

171 Athenaeus, "The Deipnosophists" (C. D. Yonge, B.A., ed.), online at http://www.perseus.tufts.edu, accessed 9 October 17.

haunted by the fear of being poisoned, probably because he had bumped off several of his close relatives with poison himself. The reputation of lemon as an antidote to poison persisted for many centuries. The English herbalist Nicholas Culpeper, in his seventeenth-century herbal, said that all citrus fruits could be used to "resist poisons."[172]

In Hindu lore lemon is used to dispel evil. Alakshmi, the sister of Lakshmi, the goddess of good fortune, is believed to bring misery and poverty. She likes sour and spicy things, so people hang lemons and chillies outside their houses and shops so that she will satisfy her hunger by eating those and leave without entering and bringing wretchedness to the inhabitants.[173]

Because the shape of a lemon resembles that of a human eye, lemons are thought to repel the evil eye by sympathetic magic. In parts of India, the evil eye is cast off by holding a lemon in each hand and waving them in a clockwise motion around the head. The lemons are then burnt on coal or immersed in flowing water to destroy the malevolent powers; the longer the lemon takes to burn, the greater the infection.[174] In Sicilian folk magic, a lemon with pins hung outside the door would repel the evil eye, while a spell to make an enemy fall ill involved taking a lemon to midnight mass on Christmas Eve, removing a bit of peel, and piercing it with pins while reciting "As many pins as I stick in this lemon, may as many ills befall you." The fruit was then thrown into a well.[175] This is similar to the spell mentioned by Charles Leland in *Aradia* (his study of Italian witchcraft in the nineteenth century), the conjuration of the lemon, which describes sticking a lemon full of coloured pins to bring good fortune or using black pins to bring ill luck.[176]

The main use of lemon is in repelling negative influences. It can be hung in the home or outside the front door, fresh or dried, to prevent negativity from entering the house. You could incorporate it into a decorative wreath with other protective herbs, such as chilli, or make the **Lemon Pomander**. Add dried lemon peel to protective sachets and charms. Use lemon juice diluted in water as a wash to purify ritual spaces, robes, and tools, or use lemon juice in the pre-ritual bath to cleanse the body and aura of negative energies. Use dried lemon peel in incense to turn away harmful magic and influences.

---

172 *Culpeper's Complete Herbal.*
173 Devdutt Pattanaik, *Devlok with Devdutt Pattanaik* (Penguin Books India, 2016).
174 https://www.hindujagruti.org/hinduism/the-evil-eye, accessed 9 October 17.
175 Elworthy, *The Evil Eye.*
176 Charles G. Leland, *Aradia: Gospel of the Witches* (Washington: Phoenix Publishing, 1990).

Though Culpeper ascribed lemon to the moon and water because of its medicinal properties,[177] it has no traditional associations with moon deities and was unknown to the ancient Egyptians, Greeks, and Romans, so any association you see with deities from those religions is spurious. Its inherent qualities do make it suitable for moon incenses and esbat use, however.

CULINARY USES

Today, lemons are a kitchen staple for most of us. Whether we use the fresh, zingy lemon zest or lemon juice, they are widely used in both sweet and savoury cooking for flavouring meat, fish, and vegetable dishes as well as desserts, pies, and tarts. Lemon is added to drinks and used to make that perennial summer favourite, **Lemonade**.

As well as adding a wonderful flavour, lemons are good for us! One lemon will provide about half your daily vitamin C needs. Before people knew about vitamins and their vital role in the body, it was a mystery why sailors developed scurvy on long voyages. In 1747 James Lind found that lemons and oranges were extremely effective at treating the disease, and the British Royal Navy ordered that its sailors should be given a daily ration of citrus juice, which led to them being known as "limeys," though it is likely that most of the fruits they consumed were lemons, rather than limes.

Be aware that the fruits you buy may be waxed, a coating to which ethanol, milk casein, or soap may have been added; ask for unwaxed lemons.

COSMETIC USES

Lemon softens the skin, diminishes wrinkles, and fades freckles and age spots. Applied well diluted to the skin, lemon juice has antibacterial and astringent properties, which helps clear blemishes, brighten dull skin, promote new cell generation, and treat oily skin and hair.

To lighten liver spots on the backs of your hands, try applying diluted lemon juice directly to the area. Leave fifteen minutes and then rinse off with warm water. Repeat daily. For another recipe, try the **Lemon Age Spot Remover** below.

To subtly lighten your hair, use a lemon hair rinse (add one tablespoon lemon juice to 500 millilitres water) and instead of rinsing it out, allow it to dry on your hair naturally. The effect will be heightened if you sit in the sun. This also treats dandruff and oily hair.

To soften the skin of knees and elbows, cut a lemon in half and sprinkle with sugar. Use this to gently scrub the area. Rinse well and moisturise.

---

177   *Culpeper's Complete Herbal.*

MEDICINAL USES

ACTIONS: antibacterial, anti-inflammatory, antioxidant, antiperiodic, antirheumatic, antiscorbutic, antiseptic, astringent, bactericide, carminative, diuretic, febrifuge, stomachic

High in vitamin C, which supports the immune system, and with antiseptic, astringent, and fever-reducing properties, lemon is a staple in the treatment of coughs and colds, and it is often added to commercial remedies. Sip **Lemon Tea** with a teaspoon of honey added or try **Lemon Cough Syrup**. Use lemon juice diluted in lukewarm water as a gargle for sore throats; the astringent juice helps shrink swollen tissue, and the acidity creates a hostile environment for viruses and bacteria. The vitamin C in lemons helps reduce the levels of histamine responsible for stuffy noses and runny eyes.

Lemon also has anti-inflammatory properties that help reduce inflammation—and therefore pain—in arthritic and rheumatic conditions, and it helps prevent the buildup of uric acid in gout. People with rheumatism and arthritis are usually told to avoid citrus fruits, but lemon, once digested, has an alkaline effect on the body. Try drinking **Lemon Tea** morning and evening.

As lemon helps to balance pH levels in the body, this makes it useful for treating stomach acidity. For heartburn, drink a glass of hot water with a teaspoon of lemon juice in it or mix ½ teaspoon of bicarbonate of soda with 1 teaspoon lemon juice in 250 millilitres (1 cup) of warm water. If you suffer from indigestion, some people find drinking **Lemon Tea** or **Lemon Barley Water** after meals helpful. As well as being caffeine-free and rich in antioxidants, lemons contain pectin fibre, which is very beneficial for colon health, plus powerful antibacterial agents. Lemon aids digestion and encourages the production of bile.

Drinking a cup of **Lemon Tea** or **Lemon Barley Water** helps to flush out toxins from the body. Many people like to drink a cup of **Lemon Tea** every morning for this purpose, but it is also a good go-to recipe for hangovers. Try **Lemon Barley Water** for urinary tract infections such as cystitis.

When you peel your lemons, do you throw away the bitter white pith? You shouldn't. It contains bioflavonoids that strengthen blood vessels and help prevent and treat arteriosclerosis and varicose veins. Include the pith in your smoothies and the health benefits will more than make up for the bitter flavour. The heart health benefits of lemons and other citrus fruits do not stop there. The pectin in citrus fruits can also help reduce cholesterol

· · · · ·

levels.[178] The vitamin C in lemons fights free radical damage and helps guard against heart disease.

Lemons contain plenty of citric acid, which reduces calcium excretion and helps prevent the formation of kidney stones.

Treat wasp stings, which are alkaline, with fresh lemon juice to neutralise them. Squeeze the juice from half a lemon and dab it on the sting. (Bee stings are acidic—use bicarbonate of soda.)

> CAUTION: Lemon is safe in food amounts and considered safe in higher medicinal amounts. However, to be on the safe side, avoid medicinal amounts during pregnancy and breastfeeding. Lemon peel may cause contact dermatitis in sensitive individuals, and applying lemon to the skin may increase the chance of sunburn. Always use lemon juice diluted, as otherwise the acid may damage tooth enamel. Those with gastro-oesophageal reflux disease may experience an increase in symptoms when consuming citrus fruit. Eating lemon peel should be avoided by those with kidney or gallbladder problems.

178   J. M. Assini, E. E. Mulvihill, and M. W. Huff, "Citrus Flavonoids and Lipid Metabolism," https://www.ncbi.nlm.nih.gov/pubmed/23254473, accessed 9 October 17. Elisabeth Wisker, Martina Daniel, and Walter Feldheim, Effects of a Fiber Concentrate from Citrus Fruits in Humans," http://www.sciencedirect.com/science/article/pii/S0271531705801757, accessed 9 October 17. G. S. Choi, et al., "Evaluation of Hesperetin 7-O-Lauryl Ether as Lipid-Lowering Agent in High-Cholesterol-Fed Rats," https://www.ncbi.nlm.nih.gov/pubmed/15186844, accessed 9 October 17.

Recipes

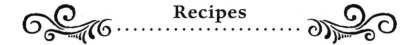

Lemon Age Spot Remover

1 TEASPOON LEMON JUICE

2 TEASPOONS VEGETABLE GLYCERINE

Combine and apply to your hands twice a day.

Lemon Tea

JUICE FROM ONE LEMON

250 MILLILITRES (1 CUP) BOILING WATER

Combine in a cup. Add honey to taste.

Lemon Pomander

LEMON

CLOVES

ORRIS ROOT POWDER

POWDERED NUTMEG (OPTIONAL)

The fruit must be fresh and unbruised. Press cloves all over into the fruit, very close together so that the flesh is not visible between them; it is best to start at the base and work upwards and round in rows. Roll the pomander in the nutmeg and powdered orris root, wrap it up in tissue paper, and put it a warm place for a few weeks until it hardens. Shake off the powder and tie a ribbon round it for hanging.

· · · · · · · · · · · · · · ·
Lemon Cough Syrup

2 LEMONS

140 MILLILITRES (½ CUP) RUNNY HONEY

60 MILLILITRES (¼ CUP) VEGETABLE GLYCERINE

Juice the lemons and strain the liquid through muslin to get a clear liquid. Add the honey and glycerine and mix together well. Bottle and refrigerate.

· · · · · · · · · · · · · · ·
Lemon Barley Water

150 GRAMS (¾ CUP) PEARL BARLEY

2 LEMONS

1½ LITRES (6 CUPS) BOILING WATER

50 GRAMS (¼ CUP) CASTER (SUPERFINE) SUGAR OR
150 MILLILITRES (½ CUP) HONEY

Put the pearl barley in a sieve and rinse well under running water. Place in a pan with the grated zest from the two lemons and the boiling water, and simmer gently for ten minutes. Remove from the heat and stir in the sugar or honey until dissolved. Cool. Strain well. Add the lemon juice to the liquid. Chill this in the fridge and serve with ice if desired. Your lemon barley water will keep in the fridge for four days. This is a traditional remedy for urinary tract infections such as cystitis, helping to flush toxins from the body, but it also helps lower cholesterol, acts as a digestive tonic, and cleanses problem skin from the inside out. (You can add the discarded pearl barley to muesli and other breakfast mixtures.)

· · · · · · ·

LEMONADE

6 LEMONS

150 GRAMS (¾ CUP) SUGAR

500 MILLILITRES (2 CUPS) BOILING WATER

500 MILLILITRES (2 CUPS) COLD WATER

HEATPROOF JUG

Juice the lemons and put the juice in a jug with the sugar. Add the boiling water and stir until the sugar has dissolved. Add the cold water and mix. Pour into bottles and refrigerate overnight. Serve with ice, mint sprigs, and lemon wedges.

Mints

Mentha spp.

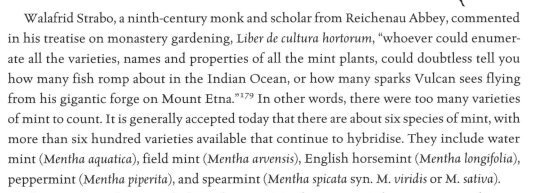

PLANETARY RULER: Venus/Mercury

ELEMENT: Air

ASSOCIATED DEITIES: Hecate, Mintha (Minthe, Menthe, Mentha), Pluto, Hades, Zeus

MAGICAL VIRTUES: Anaphrodisiac, cleansing, purification, hospitality, thought, memory, death, rebirth

Walafrid Strabo, a ninth-century monk and scholar from Reichenau Abbey, commented in his treatise on monastery gardening, *Liber de cultura hortorum*, "whoever could enumerate all the varieties, names and properties of all the mint plants, could doubtless tell you how many fish romp about in the Indian Ocean, or how many sparks Vulcan sees flying from his gigantic forge on Mount Etna."[179] In other words, there were too many varieties of mint to count. It is generally accepted today that there are about six species of mint, with more than six hundred varieties available that continue to hybridise. They include water mint (*Mentha aquatica*), field mint (*Mentha arvensis*), English horsemint (*Mentha longifolia*), peppermint (*Mentha piperita*), and spearmint (*Mentha spicata* syn. *M. viridis* or *M. sativa*).

The name *mint* has a mythological origin: Minthe was a naiad, or water nymph, associated with the river Cocytus. According to another Strabo, this time a first-century BCE Greek writer: "Near Pylus, towards the east, is a mountain named after Minthe, who,

---

179   Strabo, *On the Cultivation of Gardens*.

according to myth, became the concubine of Hades, was trampled underfoot by Kore, and was transformed into garden-mint."[180] Nearby was a temple of Hades, god of the under-world, and a grove of Demeter, Kore/Persephone's mother, who was sometimes said to have been the one to transform Minthe.

Mint and death were certainly associated in ancient Greece. It was used in funeral rites, partly because it masked the smell of decay and partly because it was an ingredient in **Kykeon**, the fermented barley drink used in Demeter and Persephone's Eleusinian mysteries, which promised a hopeful afterlife for its initiates. Try the non-alcoholic version below as a drink at the Autumn Equinox.

The Latin word *mente* means "thought" as it was believed that mint stimulated the brain. Pliny advised scholars to wear a crown made from the plant to aid concentration. Gerard said of it: "The smell of Mint does stir up the minde," and Culpeper commented: "Being smelled into, it is comfortable for the head and memory."[181]

The Roman poet Ovid wrote that mint was a symbol of hospitality and had the cordial Baucis and Philemonon scour their table with fresh mint before setting out food for the visiting gods Zeus and Hermes. Pliny recommended stuffing the cushions used at banquets with mint because "just the smell refreshes our spirits and gives zest to food."[182] Both Greeks and Romans wore mint as banquet wreaths and used it as table sprays. It was used as a strewing herb into Tudor times to freshen the air and deter mice. Gerard wrote that "the smelle rejoiceth the heart of man, for which cause they used to strew it in chambers and places of recreation, pleasure and repose, where feasts and banquets are made."[183]

Mint was thought to have a calming, if not to say sobering, effect. The followers of Bacchus, the Roman god of wine, wore mint to dispel the effects of drunkenness.[184] Aristotle and others forbade the use of mint by soldiers because it was thought to lessen or destroy their aggressiveness. It even worked as an anaphrodisiac, with Pliny warning lovers that using mint would dampen their ardour. Hippocrates believed too much mint could cause impotence.

The Hebrews used mint to purify synagogue floors, and it is mentioned as one of the consecration herbs of Solomon in the Bible. In Italy mint was strewn on the floors of

---

180   Strabo, *Geographica* VIII.3.14, online at http://penelope.uchicago.edu/Thayer/E/Roman/Texts /Strabo/8C*.html.
181   *Gerard's Herbal* and *Culpeper's Complete Herbal*.
182   Pliny the Elder, *The Natural History*.
183   *Gerard's Herbal*.
184   D'Andréa, *Ancient Herbs in the J. Paul Getty Museum Gardens*.

churches and on the ground during religious processions. As a herb of protection and puri-fication, modern witches may hang bunches of it in the home or use it in charm bags and protection amulets. **Mint Tea** can be used as a wash to cleanse the ritual area and working tools, added to the final rinse when washing robes or added to the pre-ritual bath.

Traditionally mint was gathered at dawn on Saint John's Day (Midsummer) and kept until Christmas, when folklore had it that if it was then placed on the high altar, the dried leaves would revive. Mint is one of the sacred herbs of Midsummer, and its powers are strongest when gathered on Midsummer morning. It can be dried for use later in the year or used in the food, decorations, incense, wreaths, etc., for the Midsummer rites.

Mint is a restorative, and **Peppermint Tea** can be taken after long rituals, trance work, or vision quests. It stimulates the brain, and the tea may be taken before ritual or while you are studying. **Peppermint Tea** or peppermint flower essence (see page 30) can help make you more awake and mindful so that you can understand the behavioural patterns that block your personal and spiritual growth.

Peppermint Tea can be drunk to encourage prophetic dreams. Use the tea and burn mint as an incense if you have a big decision to make while you meditate on the prospect.

CULINARY USES

Use fresh mint in salsas, dressings, pesto, and potato salads or add it to light summer soups such as pea or asparagus. Try sprinkling it over strawberries or peaches and adding it to fruit drinks, Moroccan-style sweet tea, and cocktails such as mojitos and juleps. Rub the leaves around cocktail glasses before putting in the drinks or just pop a sprig in fresh lemonade. Mint leaves can be frozen, dried, or infused in oil or vinegar.

COSMETIC USES

The Greeks and Romans used mint to scent their bathwater. In Athens each part of the body was perfumed with a different scent, and mint was used specifically on the arms.[185] Today mint is still used in beauty products and toothpaste.

Make a mint infusion by steeping several stalks of fresh mint in boiling water for twenty minutes. Pour this into the bath for a refreshing, relaxing soak, or put it in a footbath for tired feet that will leave them soft and deodorised.

Make a minty face scrub by pulverising some fresh mint and mixing it with ground oatmeal. Massage it onto your skin gently with circular motions to exfoliate, remove dead skin cells, hydrate, and moisturise your skin.

---

185   Ibid.

If your skin is oily, combine pulverised mint with honey and apply as a face pack. The vitamin A in mint helps relieve the grease and leave your skin glowing.

Use a **Mint Tea** hair rinse to reduce frizz and increase shine in your hair.

MEDICINAL USES

ACTIONS: analgesic, anti-allergic, antibacterial, antifungal, antimicrobial, antinausea, antioxidant, antiparasitic, antiseptic, antispasmodic, antiviral, carminative, cholagogue, choleretic, coolant, diaphoretic, digestive tonic, stimulant, topical anaesthetic

Of the hundreds of varieties and cultivars of the mints, peppermint (M. *piperita*) is the most used medicinally. It is a cross between water mint and spearmint.

The German Commission E (equivalent of the FDA) approves the use of fresh or dried peppermint leaf to treat spastic disorders of the gastrointestinal tract, and considers it effective in relieving gas in the digestive system. It has been used for hundreds of years for digestive problems, indigestion, bloating, wind, and nausea. **Peppermint Tea** is a common home remedy.

Mint is often added to steam baths for relieving congestion and stuffy nose. It contains menthol, a natural aromatic decongestant that helps to break up phlegm and mucus, making it easier to expel. **Peppermint Tea** cools and soothes the throat, nose and other parts of the respiratory system and helps alleviate congestion brought on by coughs and colds.

Peppermint Tea provides quick relief for nausea and may relieve headaches and migraines. You could try simply crushing some fresh mint leaves (of any variety) and rubbing them on your forehead when you feel a headache coming on.

Menthol, the compound in mint leaves that gives them their distinctive aroma, also has painkilling and anaesthetic properties. For insect bites, irritated skin, rashes, etc., bathe the affected area in **Peppermint Tea** to cool and soothe. Fresh leaves rubbed on the affected area will reduce the pain of bee and wasp stings.

Mint is a natural antimicrobial agent and breath freshener. Double-strength **Peppermint Tea** has a painkilling effect when used as a mouthwash and can help sore gums and toothache, or use it as a gargle for sore throats.

Peppermint Tea is particularly good for calming the nerves, insomnia, and anxiety.

A mild infusion acts as a sedative, whilst a stronger infusion acts as a stimulant and tonic.

CAUTION: Peppermint is considered safe in food amounts and safe for most people in medicinal amounts for up to eight weeks. Medicinal amounts should be avoided in pregnancy and if breastfeeding as it can reduce the milk flow. It should be avoided by those with gallstones, a hiatal hernia, or heartburn caused by gastroesophageal reflux disease (GERD). Peppermint should not be given to children under five. Do not take the essential oil internally. Pennyroyal (*Mentha pulegium*) is the one variety of mint that should not be taken internally or applied to the skin. It can cause serious side effects, liver and kidney damage, stomach pain, nausea, fever, confusion, restlessness, dizziness, and abortion.

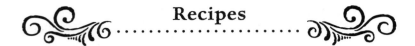

Mint Moisturiser for Combination Skin

Handful of fresh mint

250 millilitres (1 cup) boiling water

3 tablespoons coconut oil

2 tablespoons jojoba oil

1 tablespoon grapeseed oil

1 teaspoon beeswax

½ teaspoon powdered myrrh resin

Infuse the mint in boiling water for two hours. Strain and retain the liquid. Place the oils and wax in a double boiler and melt over a low heat. Separately warm the mint infusion again and dissolve the myrrh into it. Gradually add this to the oils, remove from the heat, and whisk until cool and creamy. This keeps in the fridge for up to two weeks.

Peppermint/Mint Tea

1 teaspoon dried mint or 1 tablespoon fresh

250 millilitres (1 cup) boiling water

Steep together, covered, for ten minutes. This tea, for internal use, can be made with peppermint, garden mint, spearmint, ginger mint, chocolate mint, and, indeed, most varieties of mint, but avoid pennyroyal (*Mentha pulegium*).

Peppermint Steam Inhalation

To relieve sinus congestion, put two teaspoons dried peppermint into a bowl of boiling water. Cover and allow to infuse for five minutes, remove cover, and then bend over the bowl with a towel over your head. Breathe in the warm steam for ten minutes. Peppermint is a decongestant and also has relaxing properties that can help a headache.

Minty Mouthwash

250 MILLILITRES (1 CUP) BOILING WATER

2 TEASPOONS MINT LEAVES (PEPPERMINT WORKS BEST)

1 TEASPOON FENNEL SEEDS

½ TEASPOON POWDERED MYRRH

Pour the boiling water over the other ingredients. Cover and leave to infuse twenty minutes. Strain into a clean bottle. Will keep in the fridge for two days.

Mint Liqueur

550 MILLILITRES (2½ CUPS) FRESH MINT LEAVES (WHICHEVER VARIETY YOU PREFER), SEPARATED FROM THE STEMS

850 MILLILITRES (3 CUPS) VODKA OR GIN

225 GRAMS (1 CUP PLUS 2 TABLESPOONS) WHITE SUGAR

280 MILLILITRES (1 CUP) WATER

1 TEASPOON GLYCERINE

Chop the mint leaves and pack into a glass jar. Cover them with the vodka and cover tightly. Leave in a cool place for two weeks, shaking occasionally. Strain and throw the leaves on the compost heap. Put the sugar and water in a saucepan and heat until the sugar dissolves. Remove from the heat and allow to cool completely. Combine with the minty vodka and add the glycerine. Leave for two months before bottling and one more month before drinking.

. . . .

KYKEON (NON-ALCOHOLIC VERSION)

150 GRAMS (¾ CUP) PEARL BARLEY

ZEST OF 2 LEMONS

1½ LITRES (6 CUPS) BOILING WATER

SMALL HANDFUL FRESH MINT LEAVES

150 MILLILITRES (½ CUP) HONEY

JUICE OF HALF A LEMON

Put the pearl barley in a sieve and rinse well under running water. Place in a pan with the grated zest from two lemons and the boiling water, and simmer gently for 10 minutes. Remove from the heat and stir in the mint and the honey until dissolved. Cool. Strain well. Add the lemon juice to the liquid. (You can add the discarded pearl barley to muesli and other breakfast mixtures.)

Oats

Avena sativa

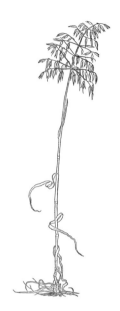

PLANETARY RULER: Venus

ELEMENT: Earth

ASSOCIATED DEITIES: Virankannos, Brighid

MAGICAL VIRTUES: Fertility, divination

A slender annual cereal with husked, drooping fruit, oats grow in temperate northern latitudes where wheat and barley struggle to mature. Archaeologists have found traces of wild oats on grinding tools from about 32,000 years ago.[186] However, though wild oats were eaten early on, they seem to have been the last of the grains to be brought into cultivation by Bronze Age farmers in northern Europe, where the climate was too cold for wheat to do well.

Oats were disparaged by the ancient Greeks and Romans as being fit only for animal fodder. Indeed, the Romans belittled the Germanic tribes as "oat-eating barbarians." Samuel Johnson (1709–1791) defined oats in his dictionary as "eaten by people in Scotland but fit only for horses in England." To which his Scottish friend and biographer James Boswell responded, "That's why England has such good horses and Scotland has such fine men!"[187] Even now, only 5 percent of the oats grown in the world are destined for human consumption.

---

186   http://www.ancient-origins.net/news-history-archaeology/stone-age-people-were-eating-porridge
      -32000-years-ago-003797, accessed 1 November 17.
187   Eric Linklater, *The Survival of Scotland* (William Heinemann, 1968).

They were certainly more valued in northern countries where growing other grains was difficult. In Nordic mythology oats are described in the *Edda* as the food of the gods.[188] The Finnish deity of oats is Virankannos (or Vironkannos), a god of growth and fertility.

Like other grains, oats are associated with abundance and used in prosperity spells. In Scandinavian countries a bundle of oats was hung by the door for good fortune. In Carpathia, as soon as a marriage ceremony was over, everybody returned to the bride's house. Before crossing the threshold, the bride and bridegroom had to pass under two loaves that were held aloft while oats were thrown and water sprinkled over the couple as a token of wealth and prosperity.[189] In Poland, on New Year's Day, oats were thrown at people to wish them wealth and prosperity.[190] In Derbyshire, in the UK, it was said that on Christmas Eve you should give a sheaf of oats to every horse, cow, or other beast about your farmhouse as an act of sympathetic magic to ensure their health during the coming year.[191]

For magic concerned with prosperity and abundance, use oats in charm bags or add them to ritual food. Hang some stalks of oats by the door to attract luck and wealth. Oats can be used in fertility magic and to convey strength and endurance. They may also be used in healing rituals and for rejuvenation and inner peace. Oats were also commonly used in money spells.

Oats were often used for divination. An old Scottish method to determine the number of children you will have is to go into an oat field at midnight, close your eyes, and pull three stalks of oats. Count the number of grains on the third stalk, and this is the number of children you will have.[192] In County Roscommon, Ireland, girls would take nine grains of oats in their mouths and, going out without speaking, walk about till they heard a man's name pronounced, and that would be the name of their future husband.[193] Such rituals are fun to try at Halloween.

On the Isle of Man, oats featured in the ritual of Bride's Bed at Candlemas (Imbolc). The mistress and servants of each family took a sheaf of oats and dressed it up in woman's apparel, put it in a large basket, and laid a wooden club by it, and this they called Briid's

188   Snorri Sturluson (Anthony Faulkes, ed.), *Edda* (W&N, New Ed edition, 2008).
189   http://www.iabsi.com/gen/under/customs%20and%20superstitions.htm, accessed 1 November 17.
190   Sophie Hodorowicz Knab, *Polish Customs, Traditions, and Folklore* (Hippocrene Books, 1996).
191   http://www.kjarrett.com/livinginthepast/2014/12/22/derbyshire-christmas-folklore-superstitions-customs-and-carols/#_edn8, accessed 7 January 18.
192   W. Grant Stewart, *The Popular Superstitions and Festive Amusements of the Highlanders of Scotland* (Edinburgh: A. Constable, 1823).
193   https://mrsdaffodildigresses.wordpress.com/2017/10/13/halloween-superstitions-ancient-times-reported-in-1916/.

· · · · ·

bed, and then the mistress and servants cried three times, "Briid is come, Briid is welcome." This they did just before going to bed, and when they rose in the morning, they looked among the ashes expecting to see the impression of Briid's club there, which, if they did, they reckoned a true omen of a good crop and a prosperous year, and if the contrary, they took it as a bad sign of things to come.[194] We always make a Brighid doll for Imbolc and enact the rite of Brighid's bed. One of the women circles the ring with the doll, saying, "Let Brighid come in," and the other women respond, "Welcome, Brigid; Brighid has come; welcome to our circle," repeating this three times. The doll is laid in a crib on the altar to represent the goddess. You can make a simple doll by taking a sheaf of oats and tying off the tops with their seeds for the head and hair, and then tie off two arms and two legs. Secure a clear quartz crystal in the body.

CULINARY USES

Oats do not contain gluten like other grains such as wheat, barley, and rye, but they are often processed near wheat, barley, and other grains, so may be contaminated; coeliac sufferers may want to avoid them unless guaranteed gluten free. The use of oats is well known in breakfast porridge, gruel, oat cakes, and haggis. **Oat Milk** is a ready replacement for cow's milk for those sensitive or adverse to dairy products.

COSMETIC USES

Skin conditions benefit greatly from oats. Ground dried oats are a traditional ingredient in cosmetics, used for their clearing and rejuvenating action. Oats contain a unique group of polyphenolics, the avenanthramides, which relieve itching, alleviate redness, and reduce inflammation and swelling. A long-chain polysaccharide, oat beta-glucan, was identified as a deep hydrating agent, capable of reducing fine lines and wrinkles, improving skin elasticity, and accelerating tissue healing,

 An oatmeal face mask will rejuvenate tired skin. You can make your own by blending oats and warm water into a paste and applying to your face; after twenty minutes rinse off with tepid water.

---

194 Moore, *The Folk-Lore of the Isle of Man.*

MEDICINAL USES

ACTIONS: antidepressant, antispasmodic, anxiolytic,
cardiotonic, demulcent, emollient, hypolipidemic, nervine,
nutritive, prostatelium, stimulant, tonic, vulnerary

Oats contain anti-inflammatory and antioxidant compounds, which many studies have found reduce the redness, dryness, scaliness, and itching of eczema. Tie a handful of oats into a square of muslin and hang from the bath tap as you run the hot water, or just drop the sachet into the bath. Bathe in the soothing water.

Oats contain a specific type of fibre known as beta-glucan that can quickly lower LDL cholesterol.[195] Studies show that just 60 to 85 grams of oats (a small bowl of porridge) a day can reduce LDL cholesterol by 8 to 23 percent,[196] or try **Maggie's Flapjacks**.

Oats contain the alkaloid gramine, which is a natural sedative.[197] To relieve stress and insomnia, oats can be included in the diet or **Oat Milk** taken before bed.

CAUTION: None known (see the note in the
culinary section about coeliac sufferers).

195   Steel (ed.), *Healing Foods.*
196   Ibid.
197   Ibid.

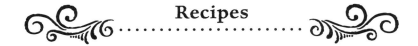

Recipes

Oat Milk

100 GRAMS (1 CUP) ROLLED OATS

1 LITRE (4 CUPS) WATER

Put in a pan, bring to boil, and reduce heat to simmer twenty minutes. Strain. Store in the fridge.

Oatcakes

115 GRAMS (1⅓ CUPS) MEDIUM OATMEAL

½ TEASPOON BICARBONATE OF SODA (BAKING SODA)

½ TEASPOON SALT

1 TEASPOON BUTTER, MELTED

HOT WATER

Mix the oatmeal, soda, and salt. Make a well in the centre and pour in the melted fat and enough hot water to make soft dough. Turn onto a surface dusted with oatmeal and form into a smooth ball. Knead and roll out thinly. Cut into eight pieces and put on a baking sheet. Bake at 180°C/350°F/gas mark 4 until the edges curl. The oatcakes should be toasted just prior to eating. These make suitable cakes for ritual, particularly if you work in the Northern Tradition.

. . . .
MAGGIE'S FLAPJACKS

150 GRAMS (2 CUPS) OATS

150 GRAMS (1 CUP) OAT FLOUR

100 GRAMS (1 CUP) ANY COMBINATION OF DRIED FRUIT, NUTS, AND SEEDS

150 GRAMS (½ CUP) HONEY

175 GRAMS (¾ CUP) MARGARINE OR BUTTER

Mix all the dry ingredients in a bowl. Gently melt the honey and margarine together in a pan or in the microwave. Add to the dry ingredients. Spoon into a baking tray. Bake for fifteen minutes at 160°C/325°F/gas mark 3. Cut while still warm.

. . . .
PROSPERITY CHARM BAG

SMALL PALM FULL OF OATS

3 ALMONDS

3 BASIL LEAVES, DRIED

1 CINNAMON STICK

7 CLOVES

PINCH OF TURMERIC POWDER

Combine in a green bag.

* * * * * * * *

OATMEAL ALE

9 LITRES (38 CUPS) WATER

1,000 GRAMS BREWING MALT EXTRACT

120 GRAMS BLACK MALT

500 GRAMS (2 CUPS) FLAKED OATS

60 GRAMS HOPS

500 GRAMS (2½ CUPS) BROWN SUGAR

STOUT YEAST AND NUTRIENT

Put half the water into a pan and bring to boil. Stir in the malt extract, black malt, oats, and hops. Cover and boil for forty-five minutes. Strain into a plastic brewing bin and put the solids into a sieve over the brewing bin. Boil the rest of the water and pour over the solids in the sieve into the brewing bin to make sure you wash out the rest of the goodness in them back into the brew. Discard the solids. Add the sugar and stir to dissolve. Cool to lukewarm. Add the yeast and nutrient, and stir well. Cover and keep in a warm place for three days. Stir and skim off scum daily. Leave to continue fermenting—this should take about a week—then siphon off into demijohns and fit airlocks. Leave in a cool place for two days. Siphon off into beer bottles, leaving four centimetres of headroom, adding ¼ teaspoon sugar to each. Seal tightly and keep in a warm place for a week, then remove to a cooler place for storage. Ready to drink after six weeks.

Oregano

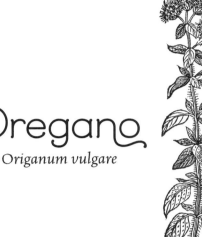

Origanum vulgare

PLANETARY RULER: Venus

ELEMENT: Air

ASSOCIATED DEITIES: Aphrodite

MAGICAL VIRTUES: Joy, love, happiness

Origanum derives from two Greek words, *oros*, meaning "mountain," and *ganos*, "joy." It is said to have been created by Aphrodite, the goddess of love herself, in order to spread happiness amongst humankind. It is native to Cyprus, Aphrodite's own island. The sweet perfume is so wonderful that it cannot help but banish sadness and inspire delight. This tells us all we need to know about oregano's primary magical powers—love, joy, and the happiness that comes from our relationships with others, whether lovers, family, or friends. In ancient Greece oregano often crowned the bride and groom, and the sheets of the marriage bed were perfumed with it.[198] Since its energy is all about delight, it can be used in all spells of love and friendship, incense, charm bags, and talismans, at handfastings and weddings and all other ceremonies of sharing and celebration.

To know joy is to banish sadness, and oregano may be used for letting go of negativity, toxic relationships, and grief. When you are working on these issues, you can drink **Oregano Tea** or anoint your body with **Oregano Infused Oil** or **Oregano Flower**

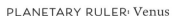

198   Watts, *Elsevier's Dictionary of Plant Lore.*

Essence, a herbal energy that specifically works on releasing past hurts, nostalgia, and the emotional baggage you carry, and relax into the flow of life in the present.

In parts of England it was said that if oregano planted on a grave flourished, it signified that the dead person was happy in the afterlife.[199] Use it in funeral incense, wreaths, or plant some on the grave of a departed loved one.

It was one of the sacred herbs gathered at Midsummer and cast on the Midsummer fires for purification. Any oregano or marjoram gathered at Midsummer was believed to be especially powerful and was kept for medicines.[200] Modern witches gather herbs Midsummer morning because at the time of greatest light they are imbued with more power. They are dried and stored for use all year round. We also put oregano into the Midsummer incense, cast it onto the bonfire, and add it to the food.

An old folk practice says if you anoint yourself with oregano before sleeping, you will dream of your future spouse.

CULINARY USES

Oregano (*Origanum vulgare*), sometimes called wild marjoram, is often confused with marjoram (*Origanum majorana* syn. *Majorana hortensis*), otherwise called sweet marjoram. Then again, oregano is sometimes just called "marjoram" in America, so the confusion is understandable. The truth is, they are related plants in the same genus and often hybridise. They look almost identical, but the scent of oregano tends to be pungent and spicy, whilst the milder-flavoured marjoram is floral and woody.

Oregano immediately brings to mind tomato sauces and Italian cooking, but it is also indispensable in the cuisines of Greece, Spain, Portugal, the Caribbean, and Mexico. It is interchangeable with marjoram in cooking, though it has a slightly stronger flavour. The aroma and taste come from the volatile oils in the plant, so always add fresh oregano near the end of cooking. Use it in salads, casseroles, soups, sauces, rice dishes, and pizzas. Oregano and marjoram both dry well and actually become sweeter when dried.

COSMETIC USES

Oregano has antifungal, antiseptic, and antioxidant properties, and is widely used in commercial medicated skin care products. It is especially useful for treating acne and pimples. If your skin is prone to breakouts, use **Oregano Tea** as a skin toner.

---

199   Watts, *Elsevier's Dictionary of Plant Lore.*
200   Ibid.

If you have an irritated, itchy, scaly scalp, the antimicrobial properties of oregano can help here too. Use a cup of **Oregano Tea** as a final hair rinse.

MEDICINAL USES

ACTIONS: antirheumatic, antiseptic, antispasmodic, antiviral, carminative, cholagogue, diaphoretic, emmenagogue, expectorant, odontalgic, parasiticide, stimulant, stomachic, tonic

The volatile oils in oregano leaves, including carvacrol, thymol, limonene, pinene, ocimene, and caryophyllene, have antiviral and antifungal properties. For vaginal thrush, add some double-strength **Oregano Tea** to the bath. For fungal nail infections, massage **Oregano Infused Oil** into the nails or soak in a bowl of water with a few drops of **Oregano Tincture** added.

The expectorant and antimicrobial activity of oregano can be useful against respiratory infections, bronchitis, and catarrh. Use the fresh herb in a facial steam and drink **Oregano Tea**. Take a cup of the tea as soon as you feel the onset of a cold or flu. Use cooled double-strength **Oregano Tea** as a gargle for sore throats or as a mouthwash.

For arthritis and rheumatism, use **Oregano Infused Oil** for a gentle massage.

CAUTION: Oregano leaf is safe when taken in the amounts found in food and safe for most people when taken by mouth or applied to the skin in medicinal amounts. Mild side effects can include stomach upset. It might also cause an allergic reaction in people who have an allergy to plants in the Lamiaceae family. Avoid medicinal amounts when pregnant or breastfeeding. Oregano might increase the risk of bleeding in people with bleeding disorders. Oregano marginally lowers blood sugar levels, so people with diabetes should use oregano cautiously and monitor blood sugar levels. It should be avoided for two weeks before surgery. Avoid if you take lithium, as larger amounts of oregano are diuretic, and this may increase the amount of lithium in your body.

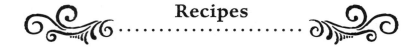

Recipes

Oregano Tea

1 TEASPOON OREGANO LEAVES

250 MILLILITRES (1 CUP) BOILING WATER

Pour the water over the herb, put on a lid, and infuse for five minutes. Strain and drink.

Oregano Infused Oil

Put bruised fresh oregano leaves in a jar and cover with vegetable oil. Put on a lid and allow to sit for two weeks, shaking the jar at least once a day. Strain through muslin into a sterilised bottle.

Oregano Tincture

Fill a jar with bruised fresh oregano and top it with enough vodka to cover. Put on a lid and allow to sit for two weeks, shaking the jar at least once a day. Strain through muslin into a sterilised bottle.

Oregano Infused Vinegar

FRESH FLOWERING TOPS OF OREGANO

CIDER VINEGAR

Put the fresh oregano, slightly bruised, into a jar. Pour on the vinegar and fit a lid. Leave to infuse three weeks in a cool, dark place. Strain through muslin into a sterilised bottle. Use diluted half and half with boiled and cooled water as a gargle for sore throats and colds. It will also help rebalance gut flora.

. . . .

Oregano Oxymel

OREGANO LEAVES

HONEY

CIDER VINEGAR

Take a sterilised jar and quarter fill it with chopped oregano leaves. Top up to half full with honey. Gently warm some cider vinegar in a pan until hand hot—do not boil or overheat. Pour the vinegar over the herbs and honey until the jar is full. Place non-metal lid (vinegar will corrode the metal and taint your oxymel). Put in a cool, dark place for two to three weeks. Now you will need to strain out the herbs, and it will help if you slightly warm the oxymel. Will keep up to one year in the fridge or six months at room temperature. Take one to two teaspoons as needed for coughs, colds, and sore throats, dissolved in warm water to taste.

. . . .

Oregano Poultice

Pound the leaves into a paste (add a little hot water to help). Apply this to the skin and cover with a warm cloth. This can be applied to relieve the pain of rheumatism, itching, and aching muscles.

. . . .

Oregano Flower Essence

Gather six to eight mature flowers. Float them on the surface of 150 millilitres spring water in a bowl and leave in the sun for three to four hours. Make sure that they are not shadowed in any way. Remove the flowers. Pour the water into a bottle and top up with 150 millilitres brandy or vodka to preserve it. This is your mother essence. To make up your flower essences for use, put seven drops from this into a 10-millilitre dropper bottle and top that up with brandy or vodka. This is your dosage bottle. The usual dose is four drops of this in a glass of water four times a day.

. . . . .

. . . .

Oregano Milk Bath

60 GRAMS (4 TABLESPOONS) POWDERED MILK

30 GRAMS (4 TABLESPOONS) CORNFLOUR (CORN STARCH)

½ TEASPOON DRIED OREGANO

½ TEASPOON DRIED ROSEMARY

½ TEASPOON DRIED SAGE

Combine the ingredients in a blender. Store in an airtight container. Add two tablespoons to your bath to ease aches and pains, uplift you, and soothe skin irritations.

. . . .

Charm Bag to Bring Joy into Your Life

OBLONG OF YELLOW CLOTH OR YELLOW BAG

1 TEASPOON OREGANO, DRIED

1 PIECE ORANGE PEEL, DRIED

7 BASIL LEAVES, DRIED

3 CARDAMOM PODS

½ TEASPOON FENNEL SEEDS

Holding your intent and wish to bring more joy and happiness into your life, sew the ingredients into a yellow-coloured bag, and carry it with you.

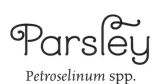 Parsley

Petroselinum spp.

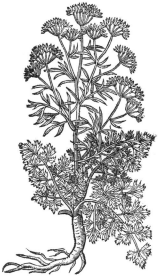

PLANETARY RULER: Mercury

ELEMENT: Air

ASSOCIATED DEITIES: Persephone, Charon, Archemoros,
Poseidon, Saint Peter, Odin, chthonic deities

MAGICAL VIRTUES: Death, funerals, underworld, spring,
rebirth, renewal

Parsley is native to the Mediterranean region, where it was a popular culinary herb in ancient times. Pliny complained that every sauce and salad contained it, and everywhere in the country sprigs of it could be found swimming in draughts of milk. The Romans are said to have used it at orgies to cover up the smell of alcohol on the breath while simultaneously aiding digestion. Pliny commented that no other plant caused such controversy because the herbalists Ghrysippus and Dionysus declared that eating parsley was a sin, as it honoured the dead at funeral feasts.[201]

In Greece and Rome it was certainly widely used as a funeral herb. The Greeks used the herb to fashion wreaths for tombs. Those people who looked as though they were at death's door were said to be "in need of parsley." Parsley is said to have sprung from the blood of Opheltes, son of the Nemean king Lycurgus. When the child was born, Lycurgus consulted the Delphic oracle to find out how he might ensure the future well-being of the

---

201 Pliny the Elder, *The Natural History.*

boy and was instructed that the child must not touch the ground until he had learned to walk. One day the infant was out with his nursemaid when they met the seven Argive generals marching against Thebes. The soldiers asked where they could find a wellspring, and the nursemaid put the child down on a bed of wet celery so she could show them. While she was away, a snake strangled Opheltes. Amphiaraus, who was a seer, interpreted this as signifying that the campaign against Thebes would be unsuccessful, so the generals held a funeral for Opheltes and instituted the Nemean Games in his honour, renaming the child Archemoros, meaning "the forerunner of death." Wreaths of parsley were used to crown the victors of the sports in these funeral games.

It has a dual meaning of death and rebirth and is sacred to Persephone, the queen of the underworld and the dead who returns to earth with the spring, bringing growth and good weather with her. Parsley is also used in the Hebrew celebration of Passover as a symbol of spring and rebirth.

One of the reasons parsley is associated with the underworld is that it is notoriously hard to germinate and very slow to come up. In England it was said that the seed goes nine times to the Devil and back before coming up, and the barren seeds the Devil keeps for himself.[202] It certainly continued to be associated with death into recent history. In England it was commonly believed that if you transplant parsley, someone in the family is sure to die.[203] It was considered such a dangerous and uncanny plant that it was surrounded by a wealth of superstitions. Some believed that only witches or the wicked could grow it, others that it was unlucky to grow it at all or you should get a stranger to plant it but never give it away. A common notion was that where it grows well, the woman is master.[204] In connection with its association with death, the best day to plant it was Good Friday, the day Jesus was executed and descended into his tomb. In Christian lore parsley was assigned to Saint Peter, who guards the gates of the afterlife.

Around 270 BCE the Greek poet Theocritus wrote of twenty beautiful maids, the pride of Greece, garlanded with wreaths of hyacinths and twining parsley on their heads at the marriage feast of King Menelaus when he married Helen. Perhaps these garlands were used to ward off evil spirits who might be jealous of the bride and groom, or perhaps the parsley presaged the bloodshed to come in the Trojan War, when Helen ran off with Paris, prince of Troy.

---

202   Iona Opie and Moira Tatem (eds.), A *Dictionary of Superstitions* (Oxford University Press, 2005).
203   Ibid.
204   Ibid.

Parsley is used by modern witches in funeral and memorial rites, whether as wreaths, offerings, in the incense, or in the food. It is also an offering to Persephone, goddess of death and rebirth with the spring. In this context it can be used as such in Ostara rituals, communication with the dead, and ancestral rites in the form of **Parsley Tea** or by being added to incense.

CULINARY USES

The most popular form of parsley is the tightly curled garden parsley (*Petroselinum crispum*), which is most often used as a garnish. Most people leave it on the side of the plate, but if they knew all the wonderful benefits of parsley, they would eat it. Parsley leaves can be finely chopped and added to salads, coleslaw, dips, sauces, salad dressings, herb butters, tomato dishes, baked potatoes, and peas. The stalks, which have a stronger flavour than the leaves, are used for flavouring casseroles and sauces. Italian parsley (*Petroselinum neapolitanum*) has deeply divided flat leaves and a much stronger taste used to flavour sauces, soups, and stews. Hamburg parsley (*Petroselinum sativum*) has large white turnip-like roots and tall, ferny leaves with a celery-like flavour. These roots can be grated into salads or soups or cooked as a vegetable.

COSMETIC USES

Parsley has antioxidant and antibacterial properties and contains high amounts of vitamin C, chlorophyll, and vitamin K. It has cleansing, purifying, toning, and lightening effects for the skin.

To relieve dark, puffy circles under your eyes, juice some parsley (or pound it up in a pestle and mortar) and apply it to the under-eye area with a cotton ball. Leave on for ten minutes and rinse. For dark patches on the face or liver spots on the hands, mix pulverised parsley and honey (you can add lemon juice for the hands) and apply as a mask. Leave it on for twenty minutes and rinse.

MEDICINAL USES

ACTIONS: antibacterial, anti-inflammatory, antioxidant, antirheumatic, aromatic, carminative, diuretic, emmenagogue, vasodilator

Parsley Tea is a natural diuretic that helps cleanse bladder infections such as cystitis. It is also useful in flushing toxins out of the system in cases of rheumatism, arthritis, and gout.

The high chlorophyll levels found in the herb have antibacterial properties that combat bad breath—just chew some fresh parsley leaves.

Poultices of parsley can be used for insect bites or you can make a salve out of the infused oil and dab on some of this. A compress of double-strength **Parsley Tea** soothes swelling and puffiness.

Parsley is rich in iron (more than any other vegetable) and vitamin C, which promotes better iron absorption and explains its role in traditional medicine for treating anaemia. If you have anaemia, you should consult a medical professional, but the rest of us can get some beneficial iron by adding fresh parsley to food.

CAUTION: No health risks have been linked to parsley when it is used for culinary purposes. No interactions between parsley and other medications are known. However, the seeds and essential oil should not be used by pregnant women, children, and people with kidney problems. Overconsumption of the seeds can lead to irritated stomach, liver, heart, and kidneys.

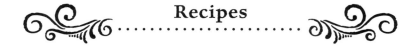

Recipes

Parsley Tea

1 TABLESPOON FRESH PARSLEY, CHOPPED, OR 1 TEASPOON DRIED PARSLEY

250 MILLILITRES (1 CUP) BOILING WATER

Pour the water over the parsley. Cover and infuse five minutes. Strain and drink.

Funeral Incense

1 PART DRIED PARSLEY

½ PART DRIED MARJORAM

½ PART DRIED OREGANO

1 PART DRIED ROSEMARY

½ PART DRIED THYME

6 PARTS MYRRH

Combine the herbs together and burn on charcoal.

Parsley Infused Oil

FRESH CHOPPED PARSLEY

VEGETABLE OIL

Put the parsley into a jar and cover with vegetable oil. Leave on a sunny windowsill for two weeks, shaking daily, and strain into a clean jar.

. . . .

Parsley Wine

450 GRAMS (7½ CUPS) FRESH PARSLEY

450 GRAMS (3 CUPS) RAISINS

RIND AND JUICE OF 2 LEMONS

RIND AND JUICE OF 2 ORANGES

900 GRAMS (4¼ CUPS) SUGAR

4½ LITRES (19 CUPS) WATER

YEAST AND NUTRIENT

Chop the parsley and place in a brewing bin. Pour the boiling water over, cover, and leave for twenty-four hours. Strain and add the raisins, lemon and orange juices, and rinds. Add half the sugar and stir to dissolve. Add the yeast and nutrient, cover and keep in a warm place for five days, stirring daily. Strain and stir in the rest of the sugar. Pour into a demijohn, fit an airlock, and leave to ferment out in a warm place. When the bubbling has stopped, syphon off into a clean demijohn, leaving the sediment behind. Fit a new airlock and leave for six to twelve months. Syphon off into sterilised bottles. This is a suitable wine for funerals and memorials.

Rosemary
Rosmarinus officinalis

PLANETARY RULER: Sun

ELEMENT: Fire

ASSOCIATED DEITIES: Aphrodite, Virgin Mary, Mnemosyne, Frau Holle, Leukothoe

MAGICAL VIRTUES: Marriage, death, remembrance, protection, exorcism, healing, love

"There's rosemary, that's for remembrance," muses Ophelia in Shakespeare's *Hamlet*. The herb has been associated with memory since ancient times. Greek and Roman students wore rosemary wreaths to help them memorise their lessons,[205] and it turns out that those ancient students were on to something. Several studies have shown that rosemary does indeed help stimulate and protect the memory. One of the compounds in rosemary oil, 1,8-cineole, is thought to act in the same way as the drugs licensed to treat dementia.[206] In 2017 the *Guardian* newspaper in the UK reported that sales of rosemary essential oil to

---

205   D'Andréa, *Ancient Herbs in the J. Paul Getty Museum Gardens.*
206   M. Moss and L. Oliver, "Plasma 1,8-Cineole Correlates with Cognitive Performance Following Exposure to Rosemary Essential Oil Aroma," *Therapeutic Advances in Psychopharmacology* 2, no. 3 (2012): 103–113. doi:10.1177/2045125312436573. Nahid Azad, et al., "Neuroprotective Effects of Carnosic Acid in an Experimental Model of Alzheimer's Disease in Rats," *Cell Journal* 13, no. 1 (spring 2011): 39–44.

students about to take exams had rocketed.[207] You can take a leaf out of their textbooks by crushing and inhaling the fresh scent of rosemary leaves while studying.

It should come as no surprise that rosemary was sacred to the goddess Mnemosyne ("Memory"), the mother of the nine Muses in Greek mythology. Storytellers and the writers of epic poetry would invoke her to help remember all the details of their tales accurately, while those about to undergo a healing sleep in the temple of Asclepius (the god of healing) would call upon her so that they might remember any visions or healing dreams while there.

It was generally believed that when the dead reached the underworld, they were confronted with the river Lethe ("Forgetfulness") and would drink from it and forget their human lives. However, initiates of the Orphic mystery schools learned that there was another river, that of Mnemosyne ("Memory"), from which they might drink and remember everything and thus attain spiritual transcendence.[208] Remembering the lessons we receive from visions, dreams, and life itself is of prime importance in our spiritual work, and in this, the energy of rosemary can help. When undertaking vision quests, dream quests, or past life work, place a sprig of rosemary by you or under your pillow, or burn an incense containing rosemary to help you recall your visions. I find a useful technique is to crush a sprig of rosemary while learning my part in a ritual, and then to carry it into the ritual: inhaling the scent brings back the words. A prayer to the goddess of memory helps too. It's a useful technique for bards and performers—apart from any magical virtue, scent is known to be a powerful memory trigger. A cup of **Rosemary Tea** before a ritual clears and concentrates the mind.

Since ancient times, rosemary has been associated with the entrance to the land of the dead, perhaps at least partly because aromatic herbs were used at funerals to mask the stench of decay, and partly because as an evergreen herb it was associated with immortality. Rosemary was customarily used in funeral rites in both Greece and Rome by being placed in the hands of the dead. The tradition of tossing rosemary into a grave prior to burial persisted through the centuries. Until early in the twentieth century, in northern Europe a sprig of rosemary was placed in the folded hands of the deceased. Mourners would also carry sprigs of rosemary to signify both death and remembering the dead. For memorial

207   Emine Saner, "Rosemary: The Mind-Bending Herb of Choice for Today's Students," https://www .theguardian.com/lifeandstyle/shortcuts/2017/may/23/rosemary-herb-choice-students-memory, accessed 22 November 17.

208   Fritz Graf and Sarah Iles Johnston, *Ritual Texts for the Afterlife: Orpheus and the Bacchic Gold Tablets* (Routlege, 2007).

rites and rituals to honour the ancestors, rosemary may be made into wreaths, carried by the participants, or added to the incense. A touching ceremony is to add rosemary to a chalice from which everyone drinks while sharing their memories of the deceased.

Rosemary was also employed to remember the vows of love and marriage. The poet Robert Herrick (1591–1674) alluded to rosemary's double meaning: "Be't for my bridall, or my buriall."[209] In the Middle Ages in Europe, the bride would wear a rosemary wreath while the groom and wedding guests wore sprigs of rosemary. At handfastings it may be included in the ritual cup, the wreaths, or the incense, and each guest might be given a bunch of rosemary tied with red ribbon to help them remember the occasion with pleasure.

The association of rosemary and love is an ancient one, and the herb appeared in many images of the Greek goddess of love, Aphrodite. According to Hesiod's *Theogony*, Aphrodite was created from the sea foam (*aphros*) produced by Uranus's genitals after his son Cronus severed them and threw them into the sea. This connection is echoed in the Latin name of the plant, *ros maris*, meaning "dew of the sea," since it thrives along Mediterranean coastlines watered by the sea mists. Rosemary can be used in spells, charm bags, and incenses for love and fidelity.

Rosemary also has the reputation of being a powerful protective plant. In Spain it was regarded as impervious to sorcery and hung over doors and windows to protect all who dwelt within,[210] while carrying a sprig averted the evil eye. It was particularly used to safeguard babies and infants; suspended over cradles, it prevented the fairies from stealing children. It was used as a strewing herb in the birthing chamber, and a sprig was used to stir the christening cup. Hang a sprig over a child's cradle to protect it. It can be used as an incense or used to cleanse a space (with a **Rosemary Smudge Stick**), and double-strength **Rosemary Tea** may be employed as a wash to cleanse the working area and magical tools. A bath to which **Rosemary Tea** is added cleanses the body, aura, and mind before ritual. To protect your home from negativity or magical attack, hang a wreath of rosemary on the front door (you will find the twigs very flexible and easy to bend into shape and secure with copper wire) and place some sprigs over the windows if you feel the need for extra protection. Carry a sprig or put some leaves into a small pouch and carry it into places where you feel someone is directing ill will against you. If you suffer from nightmares, try doing what the Romans did and place a sprig beneath your pillow. Take **Rosemary**

---

209   Robert Herrick, *Hesperides: Or, The Works Both Humane and Divine of Robert Herrick* (1856) (ReInk Books, 2018).

210   "Goddess of the Pillar: The Mythology of Upright Rosemary," http://www.paghat.com/rosemary.html, accessed 20 November 17.

Flower Essence if you feel like you are constantly battling, on edge, and worn down with the struggle. Rosemary helps you remember what is good and sacred in life so that you can find inner peace.

As well as warding off evil spirits and sorcery, it was believed to protect against disease, and as rosemary is antibacterial, this has some scientific basis. During the Great Plague of London, rosemary was carried in pouches so that the protective fragrance could be inhaled. The properties of rosemary were still being used in French hospitals up until the First World War, when an incense of rosemary and juniper was burned in sickrooms to purify the air. You can use a wash of **Rosemary Tea** to cleanse surfaces in a sick room, and use an incense of juniper and rosemary to cleanse a house in the aftermath of disease and drive out any negativity associated with it. **Rosemary Tea** may be taken to restore psychic energies after depletion and to strengthen the aura.

Finally, rosemary is an evergreen plant, its green foliage persisting through the winter. Evergreen plants are symbols of immortality, having the power to withstand death and the winter death time of the year, which is another reason it was used at funerals as a powerful representation of the survival of the spirit. In Germany it was dedicated to the crone goddess Frau Holle, and there was a legend that on Christmas Eve, at midnight, all water was changed to wine and all trees to rosemary.[211] According to medieval legends, rosemary decorating the altar at Christmas time brings special blessings to the recipients and protection against evil spirits. The wassail bowl has a sprig of rosemary in token of remembrance and it garnished the boar's head at the Christmas feast. Use it in the Yule incense and decorations and in the ritual bath, and to stir the wassail bowl or ritual cup.

CULINARY USES

I add rosemary to food as often as possible, partly because of its medical qualities but also because it is delicious and full of vitamins and minerals. It goes in soups, stews, casseroles, and is delightful in cakes and biscuits in moderation. Pop a few sprigs of rosemary in olive oil and leave for a couple of weeks to make rosemary oil (use for cooking or salad dressing) or try a few sprigs submerged in white or cider vinegar for two weeks to make rosemary vinegar for salad dressings.

---

211   Christian Rätsch and Claudia Müller-Ebeling, *Pagan Christmas* (Vermont: Inner Traditions, 2006).

COSMETIC USES

Just inhaling the scent of crushed fresh rosemary leaves lifts the spirits and has been linked to improving the mood, clearing the mind, and relieving stress.[212] An old superstition even has it that those who smell rosemary often will retain their youth; well, it's worth a try…

Rosemary is used in many commercial cosmetic products and toiletries because it has wonderful benefits for the hair and stimulates the skin, heals blemishes, and even has anti-aging properties.

I often use a cup of **Rosemary Tea** or some **Rosemary Vinegar** as a final hair rinse, which not only adds shine but stimulates hair growth and treats dandruff. It has the added advantage of gradually colouring grey hair. I rub some **Rosemary and Coconut Balm** into the ends of my hair to discourage split ends, and use it all over once a month as a deep conditioner, leaving it overnight or at least a few hours before washing my hair as usual. You can also use **Rosemary Infused Oil** as a deep conditioning oil. Warm three to four tablespoons of the oil slightly and massage into your hair and scalp. Wrap your head in a warm towel and leave on for at least an hour, then wash your hair as usual.

Rosemary is the perfect herb for a skin toner, mildly astringent and antiseptic. It was the main ingredient of the famous **Queen of Hungary Water** that, according to legend, was first prepared for Queen Isabella of Hungary during the fourteenth century. Some say that it was made for the aging queen by an alchemist, and it restored her youthfulness so well that when she was seventy she was proposed to by the twenty-five-year-old grand duke of Lithuania! The earliest recipes for this seem to be composed of rosemary and brandy and bear no relation to the various modern formulas circulating the internet, but you might like to try the version below to use as a skin toner.

MEDICINAL USES

ACTIONS: antidepressant, anti-inflammatory, antioxidant, antiseptic, antispasmodic, astringent, capillary tonic, cardiotonic, carminative, choleretic, circulatory stimulant, diaphoretic, digestive, diuretic, hepatoprotector, mild analgesic (topical), rubefacient, sedative

The specific part of the plant's name *officinalis* tells us that rosemary was included in the official pharmacopoeia because of its recognised medicinal properties.

---

212   Daniele G. Machado, "Antidepressant-like Effect of the Extract of *Rosmarinus officinalis* in Mice: Involvement of the Monoaminergic System," *Progress in Neuro-Psychopharmacology and Biological Psychiatry* 33, no. 4, (15 June 2009): 642–650.

The volatile oils in fresh rosemary leaves are strongly antiseptic. **Rosemary Tea** can be used as an antiseptic gargle or mouthwash to help heal mouth ulcers and canker sores while freshening the breath, or you can use it on the skin as a wash to clean and heal small wounds, bruises, strained muscles, and bumps.

Like most of the culinary herbs, rosemary is what herbalists call a carminative—in other words, it tones and calms the digestive system. It is particularly good for dyspepsia caused by nervous tension.

Rosemary is both a relaxant and painkiller. It is useful for migraines and tension headaches caused by tight shoulders. Drink a cup of **Rosemary Tea** when you feel a headache coming on or apply some **Rosemary Infused Oil** to your temples, neck, and shoulders.

Rosemary's anti-inflammatory and mild analgesic actions may be helpful for arthritis, rheumatic pain, and aching muscles. It contains the two powerful antioxidants and anti-inflammatory compounds called carnosol and carnosic acid, which have been shown to reduce the levels of nitric acid in the body that can be a trigger for inflammation.[213] The pain-relieving qualities of rosemary are largely the result of salicylate, a compound similar to aspirin.[214] Apply **Rosemary Infused Oil** or **Rosemary Salve** to the affected parts or put some freshly cut rosemary sprigs (along with marjoram and lavender if you like) into a cloth bag and add this to your bathwater to soothe aches. You can also use a hot compress soaked in double-strength **Rosemary Tea** applied to the painful area.

> CAUTION: Rosemary is considered safe in food amounts and safe for most people when used medicinally. Stick to food amounts if you are pregnant or breastfeeding, allergic to aspirin, have bleeding disorders, are taking blood-thinning medication, have seizure disorders, have high blood pressure, if you are taking ACE inhibitors, or if you have stomach ulcers, Crohn's disease, or ulcerative colitis. If you are diabetic, rosemary has a small lowering effect on blood sugar, so you should monitor your levels carefully. Excessively large amounts of rosemary can cause nausea or vomiting.

---

213   Daniel Poeckel et al., "Carnosic Acid and Carnosol Potently Inhibit Human 5-Lipoxygenase and Suppress Pro-Inflammatory Responses of Stimulated Human Polymorphonuclear Leukocytes," *Biochemical Pharmacology* 76, no. 1 (1 July 2008): 91–97.

214   S. J. Preston, "Comparative Analgesic and Anti-Inflammatory Properties of Sodium Salicylate and Acetylsalicylic Acid (Aspirin) in Rheumatoid Arthritis," *British Journal of Clinical Pharmacology* (May 1989).

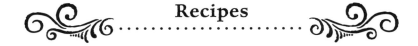

Recipes

ROSEMARY TEA

250 MILLILITRES (1 CUP) OF WATER

1 TEASPOON ROSEMARY

Bring the water to a boil. Add the rosemary herb to the water, remove from the heat, and allow it to steep for about five minutes. Strain the mixture into a teacup. Sweeten with honey.

ROSEMARY INFUSED OIL

ROSEMARY LEAVES

VEGETABLE OIL

Chop the rosemary leaves and put into a sterilised glass jar. If you are using fresh leaves, three-quarter fill the jar; if using dried leaves, quarter fill the jar. Cover with the oil and put on the lid. Leave on a sunny windowsill for two weeks, shaking daily. Strain the liquid into a clean jar. Label. This will keep for around a year in a cool, dark place.

ROSEMARY VINEGAR

ROSEMARY

CIDER VINEGAR

Half fill a jar with fresh rosemary leaves and some rosemary flowers if you have them, lightly bruised, or fill it one-quarter full with dried rosemary. Fill up the jar with cider vinegar. Leave for two to three weeks in a cool, dark place. Strain into a sterilised jar. Use as a hair rinse to add shine and condition, as a salad dressing, or add two teaspoons to warm water and drink daily to improve memory.

. . . .

ROSEMARY SALVE

ROSEMARY INFUSED OIL (SEE ABOVE)

BEESWAX, GRATED

Slightly warm your prepared oil and add the beeswax, allowing two tablespoons of grated beeswax to 500 millilitres of infused oil after the herbal material has been strained off. Pour into shallow jars to set.

. . . .

ROSEMARY FLOWER ESSENCE

Gather a few mature flowers. Float them on the surface of 150 millilitres spring water in a bowl and leave in the sun for three to four hours. Make sure that they are not shadowed in any way. Remove the flowers. Pour the water into a bottle and top up with 150 millilitres brandy or vodka to preserve it. This is your mother essence. To make up your flower essences for use, put seven drops from this into a 10-millilitre dropper bottle, and top that up with brandy or vodka. This is your dosage bottle. The usual dose is four drops of this in a glass of water four times a day. When making flower essences, it is important not to handle the flowers—it is the vibrational imprint of the flowers you want to be held by the water, not your own imprint.

. . . .

ROSEMARY AND COCONUT BALM

250 MILLILITRES (1 CUP) SOLID COCONUT OIL

HANDFUL FRESH ROSEMARY LEAVES, REMOVED
FROM THE STEM AND CHOPPED

Simmer together in a double boiler for two hours. Strain into a clean jar. To use, warm a small amount in your hands (a teaspoon or more, depending on how long your hair is), then apply to your hair and brush it in. Leave overnight (or for at least two hours) and then shampoo your hair as usual for silky locks. This also makes a good nighttime moisturiser for your skin and can be massaged into arthritic joints. It will keep for up to two years in a cool, dark place.

. . . . .

ROSEMARY SKIN TONER

5 TEASPOONS ROSEMARY

50 MILLILITRES (3 TABLESPOONS) DISTILLED WITCH HAZEL

Put the herb and witch hazel in a jar. Cover and leave for two weeks in a cool, dark place. Shake daily. Strain and use the toner after cleaning your face. This is best for oily to normal skin.

ROSEMARY AND SAGE HAIR TONIC

1 TABLESPOON ROSEMARY LEAVES

1 TABLESPOON FRESH SAGE LEAVES

250 MILLILITRES (1 CUP) BOILING WATER

250 MILLILITRES (1 CUP) CIDER VINEGAR

Put the herbs in a bowl and pour on the boiling water. Infuse until lukewarm. Strain, reserving the liquid and disposing of the herbs. Add the cider vinegar to the liquid. After washing your hair, pour on the tonic or put it into a spritzer bottle and spray it on. You can rinse your hair once more with clean water or leave the tonic on and go on to style your hair as usual. Will keep for two days in the fridge.

ROSEMARY SMUDGE STICK

ROSEMARY STEMS AND LEAVES, FRESH

COTTON STRING (DO NOT USE SYNTHETIC MATERIALS)

Gather your herbs and loosely bunch them. Begin wrapping them fairly loosely (this allows drying and also burns better when you come to use your smudge) with the string. Tie it off and trim any loose edges. Hang to dry out for around eight weeks. To use, place the smudge stick on a heatproof dish and light the end of the stick. Use the smoke for cleansing sacred spaces and auras, and for purifying sick rooms.

. . . .

QUEEN OF HUNGARY WATER

1 PART ROSES

1 PART LAVENDER

1 PART ROSEMARY

1 PART SAGE

1 PART ORANGE PEEL

1 PART LEMON PEEL

2 PARTS MINT

CIDER VINEGAR

ROSE WATER

Pack the fresh herbs into a jar and cover with cider vinegar. Leave on a sunny windowsill for two weeks, shaking daily. Strain through a coffee filter. This will keep for around a year in a cool, dark place. Dilute half and half with rose water to use as a skin toner.

. . . .

ROSEMARY ASPERGER

3 (10–20 CENTIMETRES) SPRIGS ROSEMARY

1 (10–20 CENTIMETRES) SPRIG SAGE

WHITE THREAD

1 TABLESPOON SALT

500 MILLILITRES (2 CUPS) WATER

Bind the rosemary and sage together with the white thread. Dissolve the salt in the water. Dip the rosemary and sage "wand" into the salted water and use it to sprinkle the water around spaces or tools that need to be ritually cleansed or other places that need to be cleared of negativity.

. . . . .

. . . .
Handfasting Incense

¼ PART ROSEMARY LEAVES

¼ PART CARDAMOM PODS, CRUSHED

½ PART CINNAMON POWDER

⅛ PART CLOVE, CRUSHED

¼ PART CORIANDER SEEDS, CRUSHED

⅛ PART DILL LEAVES

PINCH OF SAFFRON

4 PARTS FRANKINCENSE RESIN

Blend together and burn on charcoal.

Sage

Salvia officinalis

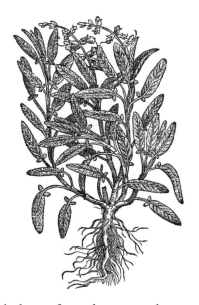

PLANETARY RULER: Jupiter

ELEMENT: Air

ASSOCIATED DEITIES: Consus, Jupiter, Zeus, Cadmus

MAGICAL VIRTUES: Healing, protection, cleansing,
purification, wisdom

The genus name Salvia and the common name *sage* both derive from the Latin *salvia*, meaning "to be in good health." The specific name *officinalis* recognised sage as a medicinal plant included in the official pharmacopoeia.

The Romans believed that its use benefited most illnesses. It was collected ritually by a priest dressed in a white tunic, barefoot, and ceremonially bathed. The sage would be cut by a tool that contained no iron after sacrifices of bread and wine were offered. Sage was dedicated to Jupiter, their chief god. The Greeks too believed that sage improved both the mind and the body and dedicated it to Zeus, their chief god. Strabo, the first-century BCE Greek geographer from Pontus, rated it first among the healthful herbs in his garden.[215] Each year the ancient Greeks offered sage leaves to the hero Cadmus, grandson of the sea god Poseidon and Nilus (the Nile River), who, according to legend, first discovered its healing virtues.[216]

---

215   Strabo, *The Geographica*.
216   D'Andréa, *Ancient Herbs in the J. Paul Getty Museum Gardens*.

In the Middle Ages sage was used to treat all kind of illnesses, from nervous complaints and palsy to fevers. According to the *Regimen Sanitatis Salernitanum* ("A Salernitan Regimen of Health") from the Salerno school of medicine, "Why should a man die in whose garden grows sage?...Sage calms the nerves, takes away hand tremors, and helps cure fever...O sage the saviour, of nature the conciliator!"[217] *Gerard's Herbal* likewise stated that sage "is singularly good for the head and brain, it quickeneth the senses and memory, strengtheneth the sinews, restoreth health to those that have the palsy, and taketh away shakey trembling of the members." An old English saying was that "He who would live for aye (ever) must eat sage in May." The French writer Saint-Simon, of the court of Louis XIV, took a tisane of it every night and attributed his long life to it.

Sage was also believed to be a great protection from illness and was sometimes called *Salvia salvatrix* ("sage the saviour") and taken to ward off plague. It was one of the ingredients of **Four Thieves Vinegar**, a blend of herbs in vinegar which was supposed to have protected a group of looters in Marseille during the Black Death. When they were caught, they offered to exchange their secret recipe in exchange for their lives.[218] Carry a sage leaf when you feel the need of protection.

All kinds of superstitions accompanied sage's use, planting, and growing. It was considered bad luck to plant sage in your own garden, so a stranger should be found to do it for you. It was also unlucky for sage to occupy a bed on its own, and it should share it with at least one other plant. It was said that if sage flourished in the garden, then business would prosper, but a withering plant indicated that business was bad. A garden where sage grows vigorously indicates the household is ruled by a strong woman.

Sage is a herb of purification. In the Bible sage is mentioned as one of the herbs that Solomon used to purify his temple, while white sage (*Salvia apianais*) is well known as a purification herb amongst the Native American peoples, used for the cleansing of mind, body, and spirit as well as sacred articles before prayers and ceremonies. You can also use garden sage in an incense or in a **Sage Smudge Stick** to cleanse the aura, the working area, and magical tools. **Sage Tea** or **Sage Purification Potion** may be used as a wash to cleanse magical tools, added to the ritual bath, or added to the water when washing robes. **Sage Tea** may be drunk whilst fasting to purify the body and spirit.

We use the word *sage* to denote a wise person or insight gained through life experience, and the plant is very much associated with wisdom; in British folklore just carrying a sage

---

217   J. Ordronaux (trans.), *Regimen Sanitatis Salerni* (Scuola Medica Salernitana), Lippincott, 1871.
218   Power and Sedgwick, *The New Sydenham Society's Lexicon of Medicine and the Allied Sciences.*

leaf was said to make you wise. You can connect with sage energy through the drinking of **Sage Tea** or by using **Sage Flower Essence** while you put aside some quiet time to meditate and listen to the quiet voice of your soul within. Working with sage energy in this way can help to align the mental and spiritual bodies, awakening spiritual interest and psychic abilities. Sage energy is especially useful if you have reached the point where you are asking yourself, "Life—what's it all about? What's the point?" and need to look at your life from another perspective in order to find answers. Drink **Sage Tea** or take four drops of **Sage Flower Essence** in a glass of water. Anoint the solar plexus chakra, the centre of inner power, with **Sage Infused Oil** or **Sage Flower Essence** as you meditate. Put a sage leaf beneath your pillow to benefit from the plant's energy as you sleep and encourage healing dreams.

Sage can also be used in incense, charm bags, and powders for spells and rituals to attract abundance.

CULINARY USES

Cooks use the leaves and stems of sage with meats, stews, soups, cheese, pasta, herb butter, and stuffings. Sage leaves and flowers can be frozen in ice cubes and added to summer drinks. Grind dried sage leaves with coarse sea salt to make a seasoning for savoury dishes.

COSMETIC USES

Sage can help keep teeth clean; try the recipe for **Sage Tooth Powder** or just rub fresh leaves onto the teeth to whiten them.

Sage is a natural disinfectant and deodoriser. Put some fresh leaves in a muslin bag or pour double-strength **Sage Tea** into the bath for an invigorating and deodorising wash. You can also make the **Sage Deodorant Spray**.

Sage contains calcium and vitamin A, which help protect the skin against the free radical damage that causes wrinkles and other signs of aging, as well as antibacterial and anti-inflammatory properties to soothe breakouts and irritated skin. Use **Sage Tea** as a skin toner. Sage used in a facial steam will tighten the pores.

Sage has traditionally been used to combat hair loss. Massage **Sage Tea** or **Sage Infused Oil** into the scalp to improve local circulation and stimulate hair growth. You can also rub **Sage Infused Oil** into your hair and scalp, wrap in a warm towel, and leave overnight or for a few hours, or use double-strength **Sage Tea** as a final hair rinse. Using sage in a hair rinse will add shine to your hair.

MEDICINAL USES

ACTIONS: astringent, antiseptic, aromatic, carminative, oestrogenic, reduces sweating, tonic, antispasmodic

Sage Tea is useful for coughs and colds, or use it double-strength as a gargle for sore throats, tonsillitis, and as a mouthwash for inflamed gums and mouth ulcers. Alternatively, take a spoonful of **Sage Electuary** when you have a cold.

Sage Tea helps menopausal women with hot flushes, night sweats, and other menopausal symptoms. Make a cup of **Sage Tea**, chill it in the fridge, and sip during the day or at the onset of a hot flush (or flash).

Sage is antiseptic. The fresh leaves can be rubbed on stings or bites, or you can use **Sage Tea** as a wash for acne, eczema, wounds, scabs, and insect bites and stings.

CAUTION: Sage is safe in food amounts or when taken medicinally short term for most people, but may be toxic when taken long term in extremely large amounts. Take care if you are diabetic (it marginally lowers blood sugar) or if you have high or low blood pressure as you may have to adjust your medication. Avoid medicinal amounts if pregnant or breastfeeding, or if you have hormone-sensitive cancers, endometriosis, uterine fibroids, seizure disorders, or take sedative medications, or for two weeks before and after surgery.

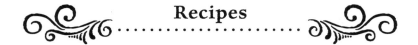

Recipes

SAGE MOUTH WASH

250 MILLILITRES (1 CUP) BOILING WATER

2 TEASPOONS DRIED SAGE

½ TEASPOON SEA SALT

Pour the boiling water over the sage. Infuse fifteen minutes. Strain. Add the sea salt to the liquid. Cool to lukewarm and use after brushing, swishing it about your mouth. Use within two days. This helps to prevent gum disease. Both sage and salt are antiseptic, reduce inflammation, and speed healing. You can also use this as a gargle for sore throats several times a day.

SAGE ELECTUARY

Pack a jar half full with sage and cover with honey—both are antibacterial. Leave to infuse two to three days or longer. Strain off the honey into a sterilised jar. Take a teaspoonful three or four times a day when you have a cough, cold, or sore throat, or dissolve a spoonful in a cup of hot water and drink.

SAGE TOOTH POWDER

2 TABLESPOONS BICARBONATE OF SODA (BAKING SODA)

½ TEASPOON SALT

¼ TEASPOON FINELY GROUND DRIED SAGE LEAVES

3 DROPS PEPPERMINT ESSENTIAL OIL

Mix the ingredients in a jar. Use to brush your teeth as normal. Will keep for up to twelve months.

. . . .

Sage Oxymel

SAGE LEAVES

HONEY

CIDER VINEGAR

Take a sterilised jar and quarter fill it with chopped sage leaves. Top up to half full with honey. Gently warm some cider vinegar in a pan until hand hot—do not boil or overheat. Pour the vinegar over the herbs and honey until the jar is full. Fit a non-metal lid (vinegar will corrode the metal and taint your oxymel). Put in a cool, dark place for two to three weeks. Strain the finished oxymel into a sterilised bottle though muslin—it will help if you slightly warm the oxymel. This will keep up to one year in the fridge or six months at room temperature. Take two teaspoons for coughs, colds, and sore throats as needed, dissolved in warm water to taste.

. . . . . .

Sage Tea

250 MILLILITRES (1 CUP) BOILING WATER

1 TEASPOON DRIED SAGE OR 2 TEASPOONS FRESH SAGE

Pour the water on the sage, cover, and infuse five minutes. Strain and drink, sweetened with honey if desired. Sip as needed during the day.

. . . .

Sage Deodorant Spray

60 MILLILITRES (¼ CUP) DISTILLED WITCH HAZEL

30 MILLILITRES (⅛ CUP) SAGE TINCTURE (SEE BELOW)

25 DROPS ESSENTIAL OILS SUCH AS LEMON OR ORANGE

Mix together in a spray bottle. Shake before use. Sage is a natural deodorant.

. . . . .

. . . .
SAGE TINCTURE

Pack a sterilised jar three-quarters full with chopped fresh sage leaves. Top up with vodka or brandy, covering the leaves well. Put on a sunny windowsill for two to three weeks, shaking daily. Strain into a clean bottle and label.

. . . .
FOUR THIEVES VINEGAR

500 MILLILITRES (2 CUPS) WHITE WINE VINEGAR

25 CLOVES, CRUSHED

3 GARLIC CLOVES, PEELED AND CRUSHED

1 TABLESPOON MARJORAM

1 TABLESPOON SAGE

1 TABLESPOON ROSEMARY

Put everything in a glass container for fifteen days, shaking daily. Strain off the vinegar into a clean bottle. This is a powerful antiseptic and disinfectant that can be used for cleaning. Add two tablespoons to your bath or use to dab on cuts and insect bites.

. . . .
SAGE FLOWER ESSENCE

Gather a few mature sage flowers. Float them on the surface of 150 millilitres spring water in a bowl and leave in the sun for three or four hours. Make sure that they are not shadowed in any way. Remove the flowers. Pour the water into a bottle and top up with 150 millilitres brandy or vodka to preserve it. This is your mother essence. To make up the sage flower essence for use, put seven drops from this into a 10-millilitre dropper bottle, and top that up with brandy or vodka. The usual dose is four drops of this in a glass of water four times a day.

. . . . .

. . . .

SAGE SMUDGE STICK

SAGE LEAVES AND FINE STEMS, DRIED

COTTON STRING (DO NOT USE SYNTHETIC MATERIALS)

Gather your herbs and loosely bunch them. Begin wrapping fairly loosely (this allows better drying and also burns better when you come to use your smudge) into a long oblong with the string. Tie it off and trim any loose edges. Hang to dry out for at least eight weeks. To use, place the smudge stick on a heatproof dish and light the end of the stick. Use the smoke for cleansing sacred spaces and auras, and for purifying sick rooms.

. . . .

SAGE PURIFICATION POTION

500 MILLILITRES (2 CUPS) BOILING WATER

3 SAGE LEAVES

7 BASIL LEAVES

3 BAY LEAVES

1 TEASPOON ROSEMARY

Pour the water over the herbs and infuse, covered, for twenty minutes. Strain and use to wash the temple, working area, and magical tools. Sprinkle around the ritual space using a sprig of fresh hyssop or rosemary. Use 250 millilitres (1 cup) in your bath when you need to be cleansed of negative energies.

. . . .

SAGE INFUSED OIL

Pack a jar with fresh sage leaves and cover with vegetable oil. Leave on a sunny windowsill for two weeks, shaking daily, then strain your oil into a clean jar.

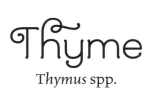

Thyme

Thymus spp.

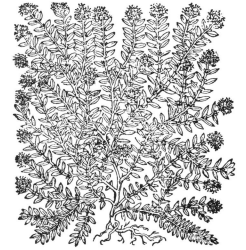

PLANETARY RULER: Venus

ELEMENT: Water

ASSOCIATED DEITIES: Ares, Mars, fairies

MAGICAL VIRTUES: Purification, fairy magic, courage, funerals, aphrodisiac, protection

During the hazy days of summer, the bees hum around the sweetly scented purple blossoms of the fragrant thyme plant. The ancient Greek writer Theophrastus observed that plentiful thyme blossoms meant a good harvest for the beekeeper,[219] while the Roman poet Ovid described the "purple hills of flowering Hymettos," where the wild thyme produced honey that was considered the best in the world.[220] Such was this association that the very idea of sweetness was associated with thyme in the classical world.

The name "thyme" is generally thought to come from the Greek for incense, *thymiama*, with an incense burner being called a *thymiaterion*, and *thuo* meaning "perfume." In both Greece and Rome, thyme was burned to produce a fragrant smoke that pleased the gods and dispelled evil. The scent of thyme was considered to be so agreeable that the phrase "to smell of thyme" meant that a person was sophisticated, self-assured, and attractive. The

---

219   D'Andréa, *Ancient Herbs in the J. Paul Getty Museum Gardens.*

220   Ovid (*Ars Amutoriu*): *Est prope purpureos collis florentis Hymetti, Fons sacer et viridi caespite mollis humus.*
       "Near the purple hills of flowering Hymettos is a sacred spring and earth soft with green grass," quoted in Burr Thompson and Griswold, *Garden Lore of Ancient Athens.*

scent was considered to be an aphrodisiac, which is why Dionysius of Syracuse strewed his palace with wild thyme before throwing one of his extravagant parties.[221] In later centuries European girls wore sprigs of thyme in their hair to make them irresistible to prospective lovers. Use thyme in potions, incense, charm bags, and powders, or wear **Thyme Infused Oil** to attract a lover. Drink **Herby Honeyed Rum** with a partner.

Others think that the name "thyme" comes from the Greek *thymos* or *thumus*, meaning "courage" or "strength,"[222] because the herb seems to not only survive but thrive when it is crushed or cut. The plant was certainly believed to invigorate warriors, and Roman soldiers bathed in thyme to give them courage and vigour, while Greek athletes anointed their chests with thyme oil before taking part in games. In mediaeval Europe thyme was an emblem of bravery, energy, and activity. Ladies gave knights gifts that included thyme leaves or embroidered a bee hovering over a sprig of thyme on a handkerchief for their warriors. Scottish Highlanders used thyme to make a drink for strength and courage. Wild thyme is the emblem of the Drummond Clan.[223] Thyme is an important herb for those following the warrior path seeking to refine their courage and their will. Take **Thyme Tea** or thyme flower essence (see page 30), or add double-strength **Thyme Tea** to a ritual bath and use dried thyme in incense to help release stress, ground yourself, focus your personal energies, and find strength within.

Thyme is also associated with death. The ancient Egyptians used it in the embalming process as a powerful antiseptic and preservative.[224] Thyme accompanied the dead in Egyptian and Etruscan funeral processions.[225] It was also used as incense and placed on coffins during funerals. The use of thyme in funerals persisted for centuries. In Wales thyme is one of the traditional herbs planted on a grave. The Order of Oddfellows still carry bunches of thyme to the funerals of members, which are thrown into the grave. You can follow these customs by planting thyme on the graves of loved ones, carrying bunches of thyme to a funeral, or adding dried thyme to the incense used at funeral and memorial services.

---

221   D'Andréa, *Ancient Herbs in the J. Paul Getty Museum Gardens.*
222   Ibid.
223   James Logan, *The Scottish Gael Or Celtic Manners as Preserved Among the Highlanders, Being an Historical and Descriptive Account of the Inhabitants, Antiquities and National Peculiarities of Scotland* (London: Smith, Elder and Comp., 1831).
224   S. S. Tawfik, M. I. Abbady, Ahmed M. Zahran, and A. M. K. Abouelalla, "Therapeutic Efficacy Attained with Thyme Essential Oil Supplementation Throughout γ-irradiated Rats," *Egypt. J. Rad. Sci. Applic.* 19, no. 1 (2006): 1–22.
225   Brunton-Seal and Seal, *Kitchen Medicine.*

In England thyme was very much associated with fairies. In Shakespeare's A *Midsummer Night's Dream*, Oberon tells Puck, "I know a bank where the wild thyme blows/Where oxlips and the nodding violet grows," because at midnight on Midsummer's night the King of the Fairies was believed to dance with his followers on wild thyme beds. It was an ingredient of many magical potions, dating from around 1600, which allowed the user to see fairies. One simple charm was to make a brew of wild thyme tops gathered near the side of a fairy hill plus grass from a fairy throne. It was an ingredient of the fairy ointment that was applied to the eyes of newborn fairy babies to enable them to see the invisible. There are several stories of human midwives accidentally getting some of the ointment in their own eyes and afterwards being able to see the fairies coming and going. However, if the fairies discovered this, they would put out the woman's eyes with a rush or stick. Like other fairy flowers, wild thyme is unlucky if brought indoors. It is one of the best herbs used to attract and work with the fairy wildfolk and in offerings, incense, and spells. When trying to make a connection with the wildfolk, drink **Thyme Tea** or thyme flower essence or anoint yourself with the **Moon and Sun Oil**. You can make an offering to the local spirits by baking some fresh thyme, rosemary, and white rose petals into a cake with oatmeal, milk, and honey, and place it in your garden or sacred place with these words: "I make this offering to honour you, spirits of this place; fill it with your power, nurture its growth, protect it, and keep it sacred."

Thyme is also a herb of purification and protection, and an infusion can be used to purify the working area. It can also be used in the ritual bath and in cleansing incenses, hung around the house, laid beneath the pillow, and placed in sachets and charm bags. Wear thyme to ward off negativity and evil. A sprig beneath the pillow keeps away nightmares.

CULINARY USES

There are many varieties of thyme, including common or garden thyme (*Thymus vulgaris*), wild thyme, also called creeping thyme or mother of thyme (*Thymus serpyllum*), and the various lemon thymes, orange thymes, and lime thyme (*Thymus citriodorus*). The leaves can be dried or preserved in vinegar or oil.

The dried or fresh leaves and flowers can be used in stews, soups, stuffings, marinades, pasta sauce, egg dishes, and with bean dishes.

COSMETIC USES

Antibacterial thyme infusion can be used as a hair rinse to combat dandruff and to stimulate hair growth. You can simply use double-strength **Thyme Tea** or try the **Thyme Anti-Dandruff Hair Rinse**.

Use in facial steams or use **Thyme Tea** as a wash for spots and acne and a natural treatment for oily skin.

Combine **Thyme Tea** with rose water or witch hazel and use as a skin toner to cleanse and tighten the skin.

MEDICINAL USES

ACTIONS: antibacterial, antifungal, antiseptic, antiviral, astringent, expectorant, secretolitic, spasmolytic

The ancient Greeks and Romans certainly used thyme medicinally. It appeared in Hippocrates' *materia medica* as a healing herb, and Pliny listed twenty-eight disorders helped by thyme remedies.

There are many varieties of thyme, but most are interchangeable medicinally. The volatile oils in thyme make it strongly antiseptic, and before the advent of modern antibiotics, oil of thyme was used to medicate bandages.[226] In fact, thymol, one of its constituents, is twenty times stronger than carbolic.[227] You can just pulp fresh thyme leaves and apply them to insect bites, cuts, and small wounds, or use double-strength **Thyme Tea** or the **Thyme Antiseptic Vinegar** as a skin wash to clean and disinfect them. Because of these antiseptic qualities, thyme is an active ingredient in various commercially produced mouthwashes such as Listerine,[228] but you can simply chew the fresh leaves or use **Thyme Tea** as a breath-freshening mouthwash or gargle that also helps relieve inflamed gums, gum disease, gingivitis, mouth ulcers, and sore throats.

Thyme is a go-to herb for coughs, colds, flu, and bronchitis. As well as stimulating the immune system and strengthening the lungs, it is an expectorant and antispasmodic, which means it helps loosen mucus so you can cough it up, and it relaxes constriction in the lungs.[229] Use the **Thyme and Lemon Tea** or **Thyme Oxymel**, or have some **Thyme**

---

226 Grieve, *A Modern Herbal*.
227 Brunton-Seal and Seal, *Kitchen Medicine*.
228 Andrea Pierce, *American Pharmaceutical Association Practical Guide to Natural Medicines* (New York: Stonesong Press, 1999).
229 Hoffman, *Medical Herbalism*.

Electuary ready for winter ailments and take a teaspoon as required. You can also add some double-strength **Thyme Tea** to your bath and inhale the scented steam.

The volatile oils of thyme are also antifungal[230] and have been shown to be effective against the various fungi that commonly infect toenails.[231] To treat fungal nail or athlete's foot (a fungal infection that grows between the toes or fingers and on nails, causing white or scaly patches, redness, and itching) use the **Thyme Antifungal Foot Soak** and let your feet soak for twenty minutes. Dry them well afterwards, as fungal infections proliferate on damp feet. Follow with **Thyme and Oregano Antifungal Foot Powder**.

Like other aromatic herbs, thyme makes a good carminative for indigestion, flatulence, and irritable bowel syndrome. Eating the raw leaves helps with the digestion of fatty foods.

A cup of **Thyme Tea** may help relieve tension headaches and hangovers.

> CAUTION: Thyme is thought to be safe for most people in food amounts
> and when taken medicinally over a short period of time. Pregnant and
> breastfeeding women should stick to food amounts to be on the safe side.
> Medicinal amounts should be avoided if you have a bleeding disorder,
> hormone-sensitive conditions such as breast, uterine, or ovarian cancer,
> endometriosis, or uterine fibroids, or if you are on anticoagulant medication.

230   Chown and Walker, *The Handmade Apothecary*.
231   Russel S. Ramsewak et al., "In Vitro Antagonistic Activity of Monoterpenes and Their Mixtures
      Against 'Toe Nail Fungus' Pathogens," *Phytotherapy Research* 17 (April 2003).

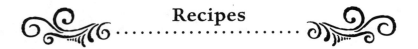

Recipes

Thyme Tea

½ TEASPOON DRIED THYME OR 1 TEASPOON FRESH THYME

250 MILLILITRES (1 CUP) BOILING WATER

Infuse together for ten minutes. Strain and drink, adding honey to taste.

Thyme and Lemon Tea

250 MILLILITRES (1 CUP) BOILING WATER

2 TEASPOONS FRESH THYME LEAVES

2 TEASPOONS HONEY

2 TEASPOONS LEMON JUICE

Pour the boiling water over the crushed thyme leaves and steep for ten minutes. Strain and stir in the honey and lemon. This is wonderful for coughs, colds, and sore throats.

Thyme Antifungal Foot Soak

300 MILLILITRES (1¼ CUPS) CIDER VINEGAR

1 LITRE (4¼ CUPS) WARM WATER

250 MILLILITRES (1 CUP) DOUBLE-STRENGTH THYME TEA

2 TABLESPOONS SALT

Combine in a foot bath or large bowl and soak your feet for about twenty minutes. Dry your feet thoroughly and follow with **Thyme and Oregano Antifungal Foot Powder**.

THYME OXYMEL

THYME LEAVES

HONEY

CIDER VINEGAR

Take a sterilised jar and quarter fill it with chopped fresh thyme leaves. Top up to half full with honey. Gently warm some cider vinegar in a pan until hand hot—do not boil or overheat. Pour the vinegar over the herbs and honey until the jar is full. Fit a non-metal lid (vinegar will corrode the metal and taint your oxymel). Put in a cool, dark place for two to three weeks. Now you will need to strain out the herbs, and it will help if you slightly warm the oxymel. It will keep up to one year in the fridge or six months at room temperature. Take two teaspoons for coughs, colds, and sore throats as needed, dissolved in warm water to taste.

THYME ELECTUARY

Put fresh thyme leaves in a glass jar to a quarter full and top up with honey. Leave in a dark place for three weeks. Strain well into a sterilised jar. Take a teaspoon as required for coughs and colds or dissolve a teaspoon of electuary into a cup of ginger tea.

HERBY HONEYED RUM

1 TEASPOON FRESH THYME LEAVES

1 TABLESPOON FRESH SAGE LEAVES

1 TABLESPOON FRESH MINT LEAVES

450 MILLILITRES (2 CUPS) DARK RUM

225 GRAMS (⅔ CUP) HONEY

Chop the herbs and cover them with the rum in a clean glass jar. Cover tightly and leave ten days. Strain, add the honey, and leave in a clean jar for another week or two before bottling. This is good for coughs and sore throats too!

. . . .

THYME ANTI-DANDRUFF HAIR RINSE

15 GRAMS (7 TABLESPOONS) DRIED SAGE LEAVES

15 GRAMS (3 TABLESPOONS) ROSEMARY LEAVES

15 GRAMS (3 TABLESPOONS) DRIED THYME

60 MILLILITRES (¼ CUP) VODKA

500 MILLILITRES (2 CUPS) CIDER VINEGAR

Put the chopped herbs, vodka, and cider vinegar in a jam jar and leave for two weeks, shaking daily. Strain into a clean jar. Shampoo your hair as normal, and add a tablespoon to the final hair rinse.

. . . .

THYME INFUSED OIL

Pack fresh thyme into a clean glass jar and cover with vegetable oil. Leave on a sunny windowsill for two weeks, shaking daily, then strain your oil into a clean jar.

. . . .

THYME ANTISEPTIC VINEGAR

HANDFUL THYME LEAVES

HANDFUL ROSEMARY LEAVES

HANDFUL SAGE LEAVES

CIDER VINEGAR OR DISTILLED WHITE VINEGAR

Roughly chop the herbs and put into a large bottle. Pour on enough vinegar to cover. Keep in a cool, dark place for two months. Strain off the herb-infused vinegar into a spritzer bottle. Use to disinfect work surfaces or small cuts and grazes.

. . . . .

. . . .

THYME AND OREGANO ANTIFUNGAL FOOT POWDER

4 TABLESPOONS DRIED AND POWDERED DRIED THYME LEAVES

4 TABLESPOONS DRIED AND POWDERED DRIED OREGANO LEAVES

½ TEASPOON POWDERED CLOVES

7 TABLESPOONS CORNFLOUR (CORNSTARCH)

7 TABLESPOONS BICARBONATE OF SODA (BAKING SODA)

20 DROPS TEA TREE ESSENTIAL OIL

Grind up the herbs in a pestle and mortar and mix in the cornstarch and bicarbonate of soda. Add the tea tree oil and mix in with the back of a metal spoon. You can put the mixture in an old talcum powder tin or a salt shaker. Apply to the feet morning, evening, and night. Cloves contain eugenol, which is an antifungal agent, while oregano and thyme contain two powerful compounds, carvacrol and thymol, which fight fungal and bacterial infections. Tea tree oil is also a powerful antifungal.

. . . .

THYME AND PEPPERMINT SORE THROAT SPRAY

1 TABLESPOON THYME TINCTURE OR GLYCERITE

1 TABLESPOON PEPPERMINT TINCTURE OR GLYCERITE

1 TABLESPOON VEGETABLE GLYCERINE

1 TABLESPOON HONEY

1 TABLESPOON CIDER VINEGAR

Blend together in a spray bottle. Spray into the back of your throat as needed. Will store for six months in the fridge.

. . . .

Thyme and Sage Sore Throat Gargle

250 MILLILITRES (1 CUP) BOILING WATER

2 TEASPOONS SAGE LEAVES

2 TEASPOONS THYME LEAVES

1 TEASPOON SALT

Pour the boiling water over the sage, thyme, and salt. Leave to infuse for thirty minutes. Strain very well through a double layer of muslin and use to gargle when you have a sore throat. Will keep two days in the fridge.

. . . .

Moon and Sun Oil

At the first waxing of the moon, take thirteen white rose petals and put them in a glass jar. Cover them with almond oil. Place the jar outside each night for three nights. Do not let the light of the sun touch it at any point. Pour off the oil into a clean jar, and bury the rose petals beneath an apple tree. Now put into the oil three hollyhock flowers, three marigold flowers, nine young leaves from a hazel, and nine sprigs of thyme. Put the jar in the sun for three days. Do not let the moonlight touch it at any point. Strain off the oil into a clean jar. Bury the herbs under an oak tree. Dab a little oil onto the third eye position in the centre of your forehead when meditating on the fairies or otherwise working with them.

Turmeric

Curcuma longa syn. C. domestica

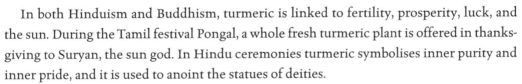

PLANETARY RULER: Sun

ELEMENT: Fire

ASSOCIATED DEITIES: Durga, Krishna, Kali, Ganesh, Suryan, Kottravai

MAGICAL VIRTUES: Fertility, prosperity, protection, purification, blessing, luck, sun, marriage, birth, death, aphrodisiac, exorcism

In both Hinduism and Buddhism, turmeric is linked to fertility, prosperity, luck, and the sun. During the Tamil festival Pongal, a whole fresh turmeric plant is offered in thanksgiving to Suryan, the sun god. In Hindu ceremonies turmeric symbolises inner purity and inner pride, and it is used to anoint the statues of deities.

The name of turmeric is synonymous with yellow in many languages, including Sanskrit.[232] In India yellow is a sacred colour, and the robes of Hindu monks were traditionally coloured with a yellow dye made of turmeric. Women apply turmeric paste to their faces to emulate the yellow glowing skin of the warrior goddess Durga, a fierce form of the protective mother goddess who battles the demonic powers that threaten peace and prosperity. Turmeric is also associated with the yellow robes of the Lord Krishna, while special Ganesh idols are made entirely of turmeric, and turmeric water is used as an offering to

---

232 Simoons, *Plants of Life, Plants of Death.*

the goddess Kali. In Buddhism, turmeric symbolises purity and prosperity and is used to anoint sacred images, as well as to dye the "saffron" robes of monks.

Because of its connection with fertility and luck, it is often used in wedding ceremonies in India. It may be applied to the bride's skin as ritual purification before the ceremony or family members apply turmeric paste to both the bride and groom in purification and blessing.[233] The bride dons a robe dyed with turmeric, and turmeric is spattered on the wall. This is to purify the couple and protect them from evil forces, foster communion between them, encourage the birth of offspring, and bring about well-being and happiness, though it also has erotic connotations.[234] A swastika (a good luck symbol in Hinduism) of turmeric is sometimes drawn on the feet of the bride and groom. In Tamil wedding ceremonies, a necklace of turmeric roots is given, and in western and coastal India, strings of turmeric tubers are tied to the wrists of the couple.[235]

Turmeric also has a reputation as an aphrodisiac. On the Marquesas it was used in quantity by adolescents during orgiastic ceremonies and other situations involving sexual activity. The smell was supposed to have a stimulating effect.[236] For the Muria of India, the yellow colour was a ghost scarer. In China turmeric was used to placate evil spirits and keep them from the house.[237] In Southeast Asia and the Pacific, turmeric is associated with crop fertility. The colour there is of paramount importance.[238] Yellow is the colour of the gods in Samoa, so the gathering and processing of turmeric roots was a sacred ceremony. It was used as a dusting powder on babies, to soothe the pain of tattooing, or rubbed on inflamed body parts.

Turmeric also plays its part in the rituals of birth and death. On the Polynesian island of Tikopia, turmeric was daubed over mother and baby as a mark of honour and used to single out individuals of special interest and importance.[239] In Bombay it was the practice to cut off the umbilical cord of a newborn child and bury it with turmeric, and elsewhere the mother is smeared with turmeric seven days after the birth, and the afterbirth is buried in a pot about which a turmeric-dyed cord has been wound.[240] Turmeric roots are often a gift to pregnant women, and turmeric's use is forbidden in a house in mourning. In southern India the dried rhizome is often worn in an amulet as protection against evil and to bring

---

233 Brahma Prakesh Pandey, *Sacred Plants of India* (New Delhi: Shree Publishing House, 1989).

234 Simoons, *Plants of Life, Plants of Death*.

235 Ibid.

236 Robert C. Suggs, *Marquesan Sexual Behaviour* (Constable, 1966).

237 Simoons, *Plants of Life, Plants of Death*.

238 Ibid.

239 Raymond Firth, *Tikopia Ritual and Belief* (Allen and Unwin, 1967).

240 Simoons, *Plants of Life, Plants of Death*.

about healing or good luck. In death rituals, a corpse might be smeared with turmeric prior to cremation. When a Hindu woman was about to commit *suttee* (suicide), she wore a cloth dyed with turmeric. The Rajputs, members of the warrior class, wore yellow robes when they went into battle heavily outnumbered and expecting to die.[241]

Turmeric is associated with luck, prosperity, and fertility. It may be used in incenses, sachets, and powders to bring luck to a home or business. It can be used at marriage or handfasting rites, in the incense, in an anointing oil, as a ritual wash before the ceremony, in the food, or in the decorations. Scatter turmeric powder on thresholds to deter evil spirits and negative energy.

CULINARY USES

Also called Indian saffron or the Golden Goddess, this perennial plant of the ginger family is native to India and South Asia. It came to the West later than many other spices. Marco Polo was among the first westerners to see it in China in 1280. He compared it to saffron in colour and scent.[242] Indeed, it is called *safran d'Inde* (Indian saffron) in French.

In commercially grown turmeric, the rhizome is dug up, cleaned, boiled, and then dried for a week in the sun before being ground into the familiar powder we buy from shops. Turmeric power is sensitive to light and should be stored in darkness.

The bright yellow powdered turmeric is well known for its use in curries and the spice blend known as curry powder. You can get more health-giving turmeric in your diet by adding it to scrambled eggs, boiled rice, soups, and smoothies.

COSMETIC USES

Indian women have known about the amazing skin care secrets of turmeric for hundreds of years. Turmeric has anti-inflammatory properties that help calm the skin and reduce redness, and its antibacterial properties combat blemishes and acne. It also improves collagen production and elasticity, stimulates new cell growth, and increases blood flow. Its healing properties combat many common skin problems. As an antioxidant, it helps tackle free radicals, which are a major factor in aging the skin. It can even reduce the appearance of dark circles and patches.

The powder can be added to face masks to clear oily skin, acne, and blemishes. Make a facial scrub for aging skin and wrinkles by adding it to ground almonds, wetting and

---

241 Ibid.
242 Brunton-Seal and Seal, *Kitchen Medicine*.

massaging on the face before rinsing, or make a turmeric face mask by combining the powder with yoghurt and honey.

One word of caution: when applied to the skin, turmeric can temporarily stain the skin yellow. This is nothing to worry about, and it will disappear with a few washes.

MEDICINAL USES

ACTIONS: alterative, anthelmintic, antibiotic, anti-inflammatory, antimicrobial, anti-platelet aggregating, antoxidant, astringent, carminative, choleretic, circulatory stimulant, hypolipidemic

Turmeric has been used in India for at least 4,000 years. In Ayurvedic medicine it is considered to promote longevity and to be a cleanser for the whole body. It is the active ingredient in **Golden Milk**, an Ayurvedic cure-all.

There have been many studies conducted over the last fifty years on the efficacy and safety of turmeric, and especially on curcumin, thought to be its most medicinally active compound. Pharmaceutical companies have introduced a new class of anti-inflammatory drugs, COX-2 inhibitors, which deliver the benefits of NSAIDs but with fewer side effects; curcumin is a natural COX-2 inhibitor.[243] Promising effects have been observed in patients with various inflammatory diseases including cancer, cardiovascular disease, arthritis, Crohn's disease, ulcerative colitis, irritable bowel disease, tropical pancreatitis, vitiligo, psoriasis, atherosclerosis, and diabetes.[244]

Turmeric is one of nature's most powerful anti-inflammatories, some studies showing it to be as effective as ibuprofen or cortisone in helping ease the stiffness and pain of arthritic joints or bursitis,[245] for which it can be externally applied as a **Turmeric Paste** or ointment or taken internally as a **Turmeric Tea**, **Golden Milk**, or **Anti-Inflammatory Turmeric Bombs**.

---

243   Ibid.
244   Subash C. Gupta, Sridevi Patchva, and Bharat B. Aggarwal, "Therapeutic Roles of Curcumin: Lessons Learned from Clinical Trials," *The AAPS Journal* 15, no. 1 (2013): 195–218.
245   Castleman, *The New Healing Herbs*.

Turmeric has also been shown to lower LDL cholesterol, even at relatively low doses. [246] Like its close relative ginger, turmeric helps thin the blood, lowers blood pressure, and prevents clotting. Using turmeric in your diet may act as a preventative agent against atherosclerosis, a condition in which fatty materials such as cholesterol accumulate and thicken the artery wall, and which may remain asymptomatic for decades.

The antioxidant and anti-inflammatory qualities of turmeric have been shown to help calm inflammatory skin conditions like eczema, scleroderma, rosacea, and psoriasis. [247] Turmeric can be added to the diet or used externally as described above.

The antiseptic and anti-inflammatory qualities of turmeric make it useful in treating small wounds. Wash well and sprinkle with turmeric powder before covering with a bandage, or make a **Turmeric Paste** with water and apply to the area.

Turmeric also has antifungal properties useful for athlete's foot and other fungal conditions. Apply **Turmeric Paste** to the affected area, and leave for twenty minutes before rinsing.

> CAUTION: Turmeric is safe in food quantities and thought to be generally safe when taken orally as a supplement or applied to the skin for up to eight months. It should not be taken in medicinal quantities when pregnant or breastfeeding, if you have gallbladder problems, bleeding disorders, or hormone-sensitive cancers, or two weeks before surgery. Avoid medicinal amounts if you have a clotting disorder or are on anti-clotting medications such as aspirin and warfarin.

---

246 I. Alwi, T. Santoso, S. Suyono, B. Sutrisna, F. D. Suyatna, S. B. Kresno, et al. "The Effect of Curcumin on Lipid Level in Patients with Acute Coronary Syndrome," *Acta Med Indones* 40, no. 4 (2008): 201–210. K. B. Soni and R. Kuttan, "Effect of Oral Curcumin Administration on Serum Peroxides and Cholesterol Levels in Human Volunteers," *Indian J Physiol Pharmacol.* 36, no. 4 (1992): 273–275.

247 https://www.psoriasis.org/treating-psoriasis/complementary-and-alternative/herbal-remedies, accessed 29 November 17.

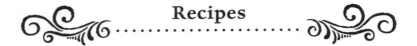

Recipes

Turmeric Electuary

3 TABLESPOONS TURMERIC POWDER

1 450-GRAM JAR RUNNY HONEY

Stir the turmeric powder into the honey. Both are antibiotic. Use on cuts and small wounds. Take half a teaspoon three times daily to fight any infection.

Turmeric Paste

30 GRAMS (3 TABLESPOONS) TURMERIC POWDER

150 MILLILITRES (⅔ CUP) WATER

Place in a pan and simmer very gently into a paste (do not boil).

Turmeric and Coconut Balm

250 MILLILITRES (1 CUP) SOLID COCONUT OIL

2 TABLESPOONS TURMERIC POWDER

Put the oil in a double boiler and add the turmeric powder. Simmer gently thirty minutes and pour into a sterilised shallow jar. Both coconut and turmeric have anti-inflammatory properties good for treating arthritis. Massage into the affected area and cover with a warm towel. Leave thirty minutes and rinse. If you wish, you can add a tablespoon of ground ginger when making the balm, which is another anti-inflammatory agent.

. . . .
Golden Milk

250 MILLILITRES (1 CUP) COCONUT MILK

1 TEASPOON TURMERIC POWDER

½ TEASPOON CINNAMON

PINCH GINGER POWDER

PINCH OF BLACK PEPPER

1 TEASPOON HONEY

Heat the milk and spices in a pan, simmering but not boiling. Remove from the heat. Leave to steep five to ten minutes. Strain into a mug and stir in the honey. The black pepper increases the absorption of turmeric in the body.

. . . .
Turmeric Tea

250 MILLILITRES (1 CUP) WATER

2 TEASPOONS TURMERIC POWDER

Bring the water to boil in a pan, add the turmeric, and boil for ten minutes. Remove from the heat and allow to cool. Drink within four hours.

. . . .
Turmeric and Ginger Tea

250 MILLILITRES (1 CUP) WATER

½ TEASPOON TURMERIC POWDER

1 INCH FRESH GINGER ROOT, PEELED AND GRATED

Bring the water to boil in a pan. Add the turmeric and ginger and simmer for about ten minutes. Strain and drink sweetened with a little honey to taste. Like turmeric, ginger contains anti-inflammatory properties.

. . . . .

· · · · · · · · · · · · · · · · ·
Turmeric Sore Throat Gargle

½ TEASPOON TURMERIC POWDER

½ TEASPOON SALT

250 MILLILITRES (1 CUP) BOILING WATER

Dissolve the turmeric powder and salt in the boiling water. Strain and allow to cool. Use to gargle several times a day to fight a sore throat. Will keep two days in the fridge.

· · · · · · · · · · · · · ·
Turmeric Face Mask

1 TEASPOON TURMERIC

1 TEASPOON HONEY

1 TEASPOON OLIVE OIL

Combine and apply to the face. Leave twenty minutes, then rinse with warm water.

· · · · · · · · · · · · · · · · ·
Anti-inflammatory Turmeric Bombs

2 TEASPOONS TURMERIC POWDER

1 TABLESPOON SET HONEY

½ TEASPOON BLACK PEPPER

1 TEASPOON COCONUT OIL

2 TABLESPOONS GROUND ALMONDS

Mix the ingredients together to form a stiff paste. Shape into small balls and then you can roll them in ground nuts, seeds, or cocoa powder. Store in the fridge for up to four weeks. Eat one or two a day.

. . . .

Good Luck Charm Bag

AN OBLONG OF ORANGE CLOTH OR AN ORANGE BAG

1 TEASPOON TURMERIC POWDER OR 1 CENTIMETRE DRIED TURMERIC ROOT

1 WHOLE NUTMEG

1 TEASPOON OREGANO, DRIED

3 BASIL LEAVES, DRIED

Sew the ingredients into an orange bag, holding your intent in your mind as you do so.

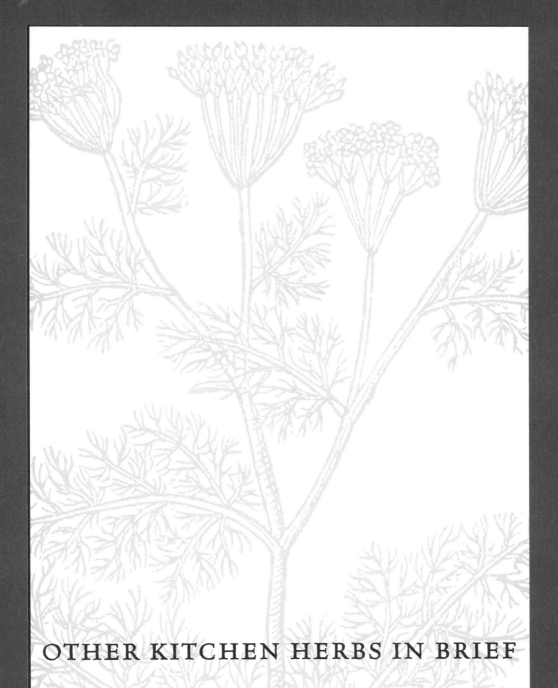

OTHER KITCHEN HERBS IN BRIEF

ALFALFA (*MEDICAGO SATIVA*): *Medicinal*—nutritive, diuretic, lowers cholesterol, digestive, laxative, tonic, anti-inflammatory. **Caution:** avoid if you are on warfarin or have an auto-immune disease. *Magical*—grounding, money, prosperity, protection. Ruled by the planet Venus and the element of earth.

ALLSPICE (*PIMENTA DIOICA*): *Medicinal*—antibacterial, hypotensive, antineuralgic, analgesic, antitumour, carminative, digestive stimulant, aromatic, anti-inflammatory, rubefacient, antiflatulent. **Caution:** avoid for two weeks before surgery. *Magical*—energy, healing, luck, money, virility. Ruled by the planet Mars and the element of fire.

ALMOND (*PRUNUS DULCIS* SYN. *PRUNUS AMYGDALUS/AMYGDALUS COMMUNIS/AMYGDALUS DULCIS*): *Medicinal*—hypoglycaemic, lowers LDL and total cholesterol levels, immunostimulant, antioxidant, hepato-protective. *Magical*—Ostara, regeneration, divination, fertility, love, luck, money. Ruled by the planets Mercury and the sun and the element of air. Sacred to Zeus, Freya, Phyllis, Amacas, Demophoon, Cybele, Attis, Nana, Car, Metis, Carmenta, and the Caryatids.

AMARANTH (*AMARANTHUS* SPP.): *Medicinal*—astringent, antioxidant, lowers cholesterol. *Magical*—death, funerals, healing, immortality, protection. Sacred to Artemis and Demeter. It is ruled by the planet Saturn and the element of fire.

ANGELICA (*ANGELICA ARCHANGELICA* SYN. *ANGELICA OFFICINALIS*): *Medicinal*—expectorant, carminative, bitter, bactericidal, circulatory stimulant, antioxidant. **Caution:** avoid if pregnant or breastfeeding, or if you take warfarin. *Magical*—Beltane, Midsummer, healing, protection, cleansing, exorcism, purification, banishing, blessing, clairvoyance, visions, warding, peace. Ruled by the sun and the element of fire. Sacred to sun gods and Venus.

ANISE (*PIMPINELLA ANISUM*): *Medicinal*—digestive, carminative, aromatic, galactogogue, diaphoretic. **Caution:** avoid if you have any condition that might be made worse by exposure to oestrogen. *Magical*—clairvoyance, banishing, divination, exorcism, protection. Ruled by the planet Mercury and the element of air. Sacred to Apollo, Hermes, and Mercury.

APPLE (*MALUS* SPP.): *Medicinal*—antioxidant, hypolipidemic, hypotensive. *Magical*—fertility, lust, love, marriage, immortality, fidelity, harvest, initiation, wisdom. Ruled by the sun and Venus and the element of water. Sacred to Aphrodite, Apollo, Bel, Ceridwen, Demeter, Diana, Eve, Flora, Godiva, Herakles, Hesperides, Iduna, Inanna, Kore, Lugh, Mêliae, Morgana, Nehallenia, Olwen, Persephone, Pomona, sun gods, Titaea, Venus, and Zeus.

APRICOT (*PRUNUS ARMENIACA*): *Medicinal*—the fruit is a mild laxative and is cleansing. *Magical*—love. Ruled by the planet Venus and the element of water.

ARROWROOT (*MARANTA ARUNDINACEAE*): *Medicinal*—demulcent, anti-inflammatory, antiseptic. *Magical*—good luck, prosperity. Ruled by the planet Jupiter and the element of water.

ASAFOETIDA (*FERULA FOETIDA*): *Medicinal*—antispasmodic, expectorant, stimulant, emmenagogue, vermifuge, sedative, hypotensive. **Caution:** should not be taken by children, if pregnant or breastfeeding, or if you have bleeding disorders, gastro-intestinal problems, or blood pressure problems. *Magical*—exorcism, purification, prophetic dreams, fertility. Ruled by Saturn or Mars and the element of fire. Sacred to Athene, Priapus, and Saturn.

ASPARAGUS (*ASPARAGUS OFFICINALIS*): *Medicinal*—antispasmodic, aperient, cardiac, demulcent, diaphoretic, diuretic, sedative, tonic. *Magical*—fertility, lust, potency. Ruled by the planets Mars and Jupiter, the element of fire, and the signs Gemini and Virgo. Sacred to Zeus, Hermes, and Mercury.

AVOCADO (*PERSEA AMERICANA*): *Medicinal*—nutritive, lowers cholesterol levels, antioxidant, antimicrobial. *Magical*—happiness, wealth, longevity, love, lust.

BARLEY (*HORDEUM VULGARE*): *Medicinal*—diuretic, demulcent, expectorant, galactofuge, lenitive, stomachic, digestive, emollient, nutritive, febrifuge, stomachic. **Caution:** best avoided by nursing mothers since it can reduce milk flow. *Magical*—fertility, initiation, harvest, Lughnasa, and the Autumn Equinox. Sacred to Demeter and Ceres.

· · · · ·

BAY (*LAURUS NOBILIS*): *Medicinal*—external use as a compress on bruises and sprains. **Caution:** avoid if pregnant. *Magical*—prophecy, divination, healing, consecrating tarot cards, protection, banishing negativity, cleansing, spiritual purification, prophetic dreams, sealing. Ruled by the sun and the element of fire. Sacred to gods of healing, Adonis, Apollo, Aesculapius, Ceres, Ceridwen, Cupid, Daphne, Eros, Faunus, Ra, Vishnu, Mars, Ares, and sun and dawn gods and goddesses.

BERGAMOT, MONARDA (*MONARDA DIDYMA*): *Medicinal*—anthelmintic, carminative, diuretic, expectorant, febrifuge, rubefacient, stimulant. **Caution:** avoid if pregnant or breastfeeding. *Magical*—protection, meditation. Ruled by the planet Mercury and the element of air.

BERGAMOT, CITRUS (*CITRUS BERGAMIA*): *Medicinal*—carminative, antiseptic, antispasmodic. *Magical*—money and success. Ruled by the planet Mercury and the element of air.

BILBERRY (*VACCINIUM MYRTILLUS*): *Medicinal*—antioxidant, gastro-intestinal, anti-inflammatory, antioedematous, vasoprotective. *Magical*—counter magic, protection, luck, money. Ruled by the planet Jupiter and the elements fire and water.

BLACKBERRY (*RUBUS FRUCTICOSUS*): *Medicinal*—astringent, depurative, diuretic, tonic, vulnerary. *Magical*—Autumn Equinox, harvest, abundance, death, consecrating the cup or cauldron. Ruled by the planet Venus and the element of water. Sacred to Brigantia, Brighid, fairies, and harvest goddesses.

BLUEBERRY (*VACCINIUM CORYMBOSUM*): *Medicinal*—nutritive, antioxidant, astringent, anti-inflammatory, circulatory stimulant, hypotensive. *Magical*—protection and counter magic. Ruled by the planet Jupiter and the element of water.

BUCKWHEAT (*FAGOPYRUM ESCULENTUM*): *Medicinal*—anti-inflammatory, antioxidant, demulcent, diuretic, nutritive, tonic, vasodilator, antihistamine. *Magical*—protection from negativity, poverty, and evil; money attraction and wealth; Autumn Equinox. Ruled by the planet Venus and the element of earth. Sacred to harvest gods and goddesses.

CABBAGE (*BRASSICA OLERACEA*): *Medicinal*—used externally as a cooling, soothing poultice for inflamed and irritated skin. *Magical*—luck. Ruled by the moon and the element of water.

CAROB (*CERATONIA SILIQUA*): *Medicinal*—mild laxative. *Magical*—health, wealth. Ruled by the planet Jupiter and the element of fire. Sacred to Zeus and Jupiter.

CHERRY (*PRUNUS AVIUM*): *Medicinal*—astringent, diuretic, tonic. *Magical*—happiness, love, divination.

CHERVIL (*ANTHRISCUS CEREFOLIUM*): *Medicinal*—tonic, digestive, diuretic, expectorant, stimulant. **Caution:** avoid if pregnant or breastfeeding. *Magical*—mental activity, clarity, Samhain, initiation, connection to the higher self. Ruled by the planet Jupiter and the elements of air and water. Sacred to the goddess Ceridwen.

CHICORY (*CICHORIUM INTYBUS*): *Medicinal*—liver tonic, bitter, laxative, mild diuretic, anti-inflammatory. **Caution:** avoid medicinal use if pregnant or breastfeeding. *Magical*—removal of obstacles, invisibility, Lughnasa, Autumn Equinox. Ruled by Jupiter and the element of air. Sacred to harvest gods and goddesses.

CLARY SAGE (*SALVIA SCLAREA*): *Medicinal*—antispasmodic, appetizer, aromatic, astringent, balsamic, carminative, pectoral, tonic. **Caution:** avoid if you are taking chloral hydrate or hexobarbitone. *Magical*—visions, getting the sight, opening the third eye. Ruled by Mercury and the moon and the element of air.

COCONUT (*COCOS NUCIFERA*): *Medicinal*—antiviral, antibacterial, antifungal. *Magical*—luck, purification, protection, chastity.

CORN (I.E., ALL GRAIN CROPS): *Magical*—abundance, harvest, Autumn Equinox, Lughnasa. Ruled by the sun and the element of fire. Sacred to gods and goddesses of the harvest such as Demeter and Ceres.

CUCUMBER (*CUCUMIS SATIVUS*): *Medicinal*—depurative, diuretic, emollient, purgative, resolvent. *Magical*—chastity, healing, fertility, astral travel. Ruled by the moon and the element of water.

DATE PALM (*PHOENIX DACTYLIFERA*): *Medicinal*—nutritive, laxative. *Magical*—regeneration, fertility, rebirth. Sacred to Amun, Isis, Lat, Demeter, Leto, Nike, Inanna, and Nepthys.

FIG (*FICUS CARICA*): *Medicinal*—laxative. *Magical*—love, fertility. Ruled by the planet Jupiter and the element of fire. Sacred to Dionysus, Bacchus, Juno, Pan, and Isis.

FRANGIPANI (*PLUMERIA* SPP.): *Medicinal*—antipyretic, antibiotic. *Magical*—love, attraction.

• • • • •

HAZEL (*CORYLUS AVELLANA*): *Medicinal*—astringent, diaphoretic, febrifuge, nutritive, odontalgic, stomachic, tonic. *Magical*—Autumn Equinox, wisdom, inspiration, making and consecrating wands, dowsing, protection. Ruled by the planet Mercury and the element of air. Sacred to Aengus, Artemis, Diana, Chandra, Connla, Fionn, Hecate, Lleu, Lugh, Mac Coll, Manannan, Mercury, Ogma, Taliesin, Thor, and Boann.

HIBISCUS (*HIBISCUS* SPP.): *Medicinal*—anti-inflammatory, hypotensive, lowers LDL cholesterol, antioxidant, antibacterial, diuretic. **Caution:** avoid medicinal use if you have low blood pressure or are pregnant or breastfeeding. *Magical*—love, lust, divination.

HOP (*HUMULUS LUPULUS*): *Medicinal*—anaphrodisiac, analgesic, antiseptic, antispasmodic, anodyne, astringent, bitter, diuretic, febrifuge, hypnotic, nervine, sedative, stimulant, stomachic, tonic, vermifuge. *Magical*—Lughnasa, underworld travel, wolf totems. Ruled by the planet Mars and the element of air. Sacred to Brighid and Leto.

LIME (*CITRUS ACIDA*): *Medicinal*—nutritive, antiscorbutic, antiviral, tonic, astringent, antiseptic, antibacterial. *Magical*—healing, love, protection. Ruled by the element of fire.

NUTMEG (*MYRISTICA FRAGRANS*): *Medicinal*—sedative, carminative, aromatic, antispasmodic, antimicrobial, antiemetic, hypotensive. **Caution:** avoid if pregnant or breastfeeding. *Magical*—counter magic, luck, justice, money, virility, aphrodisiac, Yule. Ruled by the planet Jupiter and the element of air.

OLIVE (*OLEA EUROPAEA*): *Medicinal*—antioxidant, bitter tonic, hypotensive. *Magical*—new beginnings, peace, continuity, the expulsion of evil and negativity, consecration, purification, blessing. Ruled by the sun and the element of fire. Sacred to Amun Ra, Apollo, Artemis, Athene, Auxesia Hera, Damia, Demeter, Ganymede, Hercules, Hermes, Indra, Isis, Juno, Jupiter, Nut, Poseidon, sun gods, and Zeus.

ONION (*ALLIUM CEPA*): *Medicinal*—antimicrobial, antibiotic, antibacterial, antifungal, anticoagulant, antidiabetic, anti-inflammatory, antimutagenic. *Magical*—protection, dispelling negativity, exorcism. Ruled by the planet Mars and the element of fire.

ORANGE (*CITRUS × SINENSIS*): *Medicinal*—antioxidants, appetizer, astringent, blood purifier. *Magical*—love, energy, joy. Ruled by the sun and the element of fire.

PEAR (*PYRUS COMMUNIS*): *Medicinal*—anti-inflammatory, antioxidant, nutritive. *Magical*—love, marriage, fertility. Ruled by the planet Venus and the element of water. Sacred to Hera and Juno.

RUE (*RUTA GRAVEOLENS*): *Medicinal*—anthelmintic, antidote, antispasmodic, carminative, emetic, emmenagogue, expectorant, haemostatic, ophthalmic, rubefacient, strongly stimulant, mildly stomachic, uterotonic. **Caution:** Rue is generally safe in food amounts but is not recommended in medicinal quantities. Avoid if you are pregnant or breastfeeding. *Magical*—anaphrodisiac, inner vision, clairvoyance, banishes negative energies, exorcism, purification. It is ruled by the sun and the element of fire. Sacred to Aradia, Diana, Hermes, Horus, Mars, Menthu, Mercury, and Odysseus.

SAFFRON (*CROCUS SATIVUS*): *Medicinal*—anodyne, antispasmodic, aphrodisiac, appetizer, carminative, diaphoretic, emmenagogue, expectorant, sedative, stimulant. **Caution:** avoid large amounts in pregnancy and breastfeeding or if you have bipolar disorder, a heart condition, or low blood pressure. *Magical*—love, marriage, handfasting, lifts the spirits, divination, aphrodisiac, beginnings, dawn, strength, wealth. Though given to the sun by the astrologer-herbalists, for its golden stamens and dye, the ancients thought saffron was sacred to moon goddesses. It is ruled by the sun and the element of fire. Sacred to the deities Amun Ra, Ashtoreth, Eos, Indra, Jupiter, and Zeus.

SORREL (*RUMEX ACETOSA*): *Medicinal*—stringent, diuretic, laxative, refrigerant. **Caution:** avoid large amounts if you have kidney stones or kidney disease and during pregnancy and breastfeeding. It should not be taken by children. *Magical*—love. Ruled by the planet Venus and the element of earth. Sacred to Venus and Aphrodite.

STAR ANISE (*ILLICIUM VERUM*): *Medicinal*—antiviral, antifungal, antibacterial, antioxidant. *Magical*—psychic skills, protection, prosperity, ritual cleansing. Ruled by the planet Jupiter and the element of air.

STRAWBERRY (*FRAGARIA* SPP.): *Medicinal*—mildly astringent, diuretic, laxative, tonic. *Magical*—blessing, love, Midsummer, fertility. Ruled by the planet Venus and the elements of earth or water. Sacred to fairies, Freya, love goddesses, and mother goddesses.

· · · · ·

TANGERINE (*CITRUS TANGERINA*): *Medicinal*—antioxidant, anti-inflammatory, antiseptic, depurative, sedative, stomachic, antispasmodic, tonic, digestive. *Magical*—energy, strength, power. Ruled by the sun and the element of fire.

TEA (*CAMELLIA SINENSIS*): *Medicinal*—stimulant, astringent, antioxidant. *Magical*—courage, strength, prosperity. Ruled by the sun and the element of fire.

TOMATO (*SOLANUM LYCOPERSICUM*): *Medicinal*—antioxidant, anti-inflammatory. *Magical*—love, protection.

VANILLA (*VANILLA PLANIFOLIA*): *Medicinal*—antioxidant, anti-inflammatory. *Magical*—happiness, good fortune.

VINE, GRAPE (*VITIS VINAFERA*): *Medicinal*—vasoprotective, venotonic, antioxidant, astringent, collagen stabilising. *Magical*—everlasting life, divine intoxication, entheogen, negating the ego, Lughnasa and the Autumn Equinox. Ruled by the sun and the element of fire. Sacred to Adonis, Apollo, Bacchus, Dionysus, Flora, Inanna, Ishtar, Liber Pater, Orpheus, Osiris, and Ra.

WALNUT (*JUGLANS REGIA*): *Medicinal*—antilithic, diuretic, stimulant. *Magical*—fertility, anointing, wishes. Ruled by the sun and the element of fire. Sacred to Adonis, Apollo, and Jupiter.

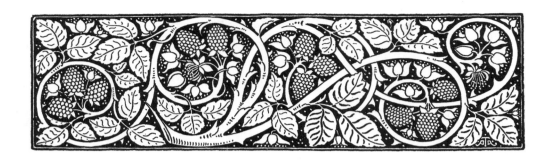

Kitchen Herb Magical Correspondences

* * *

LOVE

Apple Apricot Basil Bay Caraway Cardamom
Cinnamon Clove Coriander Cumin Dill Fenugreek
Ginger Hazel Lemon Oats Orange Oregano
Poppy Seeds Rosemary Saffron Thyme Vanilla

APHRODISIACS

Caraway Cardamom Cinnamon Clove Coriander
Cumin Garlic Ginger

Anaphrodisiacs

Hops   Marjoram   Peppermint

Handfasting

Anise   Apple   Cardamom   Cinnamon   Clove   Coriander   Dill
Marjoram   Rosemary   Rue   Saffron   Sorrel   Strawberry

Fidelity

Caraway   Cumin

Funerals and Mourning

Basil   Caraway   Garlic   Marjoram   Oregano   Parsley   Rosemary   Thyme

Protection

Asafoetida   Basil   Bay   Black Pepper   Caraway   Chilli
Cinnamon   Clove   Coriander   Dill   Fennel   Fenugreek
Garlic   Ginger   Lemon   Marjoram   Onion   Oregano   Parsley
Rosemary   Rue   Sage   Thyme   Turmeric

Cleansing and Purification

Anise   Basil   Bay   Bean   Caraway   Clove   Coconut   Dill
Fennel   Garlic   Juniper   Lemon   Mint   Parsley
Peppermint   Rosemary   Rue   Sage   Thyme

Dispelling Negative Influences

Basil   Black Pepper   Chilli   Clove   Dill   Fenugreek   Garlic   Lemon

Psychic Awareness

Angelica   Anise   Basil   Bay   Chilli   Cinnamon

AURA CLEANSING

Angelica   Bean   Rosemary   Sage

HEALING

Allspice   Apple   Basil   Bay   Black Pepper   Cinnamon   Citron
Fennel   Garlic   Juniper   Lime   Mint   Peppermint
Rosemary   Sage   Spearmint   Thyme

DIVINATION

Anise   Bay   Chicory   Cinnamon   Mace   Nutmeg

CONSECRATION

Bay   Caraway   Chicory   Mint   Olive   Rue

EXORCISM

Asafoetida   Basil   Beans   Black Pepper
Chilli   Clove   Cumin   Garlic   Juniper   Mint   Rosemary   Rue

PROSPERITY

Allspice   Almond   Basil   Cinnamon   Clove   Dill   Fenugreek
Ginger   Mint   Nutmeg   Oats   Orange   Rice   Turmeric   Wheat

LUCK

Basil   Clove   Turmeric

RETENTION

Caraway   Cumin

EARTH (ELEMENT)

Alfalfa   Barley   Buckwheat   Rhubarb   Sage   Sorrel   Tonka Bean

AIR (ELEMENT)

Almond   Anise   Bean   Caraway   Celery   Chervil   Chicory   Dill
Fenugreek   Hazel   Hop   Marjoram   Mint   Nutmeg   Parsley   Sage

FIRE (ELEMENT)

Angelica   Asafoetida   Basil   Bay   Cinnamon   Clove   Coriander   Dill
Fennel   Garlic   Gorse   Horseradish   Juniper   Mustard
Olive   Orange   Rosemary   Rue   Saffron   Tarragon   Vine (Grape)   Walnut

WATER (ELEMENT)

Apple   Cardamom   Melon   Poppy Seeds   Thyme   Vanilla

SUN (PLANET)

Angelica   Bay   Caraway   Cinnamon   Citron   Clove   Grape
Juniper   Olive   Orange   Rosemary   Rue   Saffron   Walnut

MOON (PLANET)

Lemon   Melon   Poppy Seeds

MERCURY (PLANET)

Almond   Anise   Bean   Caraway   Celery   Dill   Fennel
Fenugreek   Hazel   Marjoram   Parsley   Peppermint   Spearmint

VENUS (PLANET)

Alfalfa   Apple   Blackberry   Buckwheat   Cardamom
Mint   Sorrel   Strawberry   Thyme   Vanilla

MARS (PLANET)

Allspice   Asafoetida   Basil   Black Pepper   Coffee   Coriander
Galangal   Garlic   Ginger   Horseradish   Juniper   Mustard
Onion   Pennyroyal   Rue   Tarragon

JUPITER (PLANET)

Agrimony   Chervil   Chicory   Clove   Mace   Nutmeg   Sage   Star Anise

SATURN (PLANET)

Asafoetida   Amaranth

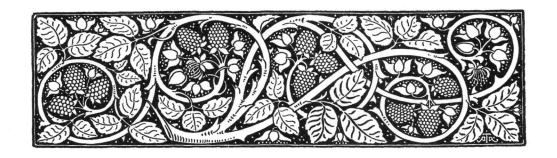

Colour Correspondences

BLACK: banishing, repelling, death, endings, destruction, winding down, the elderly, ancestor contact, the void or womb, receptivity, reincarnation, rejection of ego, possibilities waiting to be realised, Samhain, crone goddesses and death deities, the planet Saturn, Scorpio and Capricorn.

BLUE: tranquillity, peace, calm, harmony, protection, healing, spiritual development, teaching, luck, Autumn Equinox, spiritual protection, throat chakra, moon, water spirits, the planet Jupiter, the element of water, Virgo and Aquarius.

BROWN: grounding, stability, earthiness, sexuality, practicality, environmental awareness, the planet Earth, Autumn Equinox, Mother Earth and nature deities.

GOLD: happiness, rejuvenation, spiritual strength, spiritual zest, service to others, friendship, healing, energy, spiritual energy, strength, life force, solar plexus chakra, sun and corn deities, Midsummer, the sun.

GREEN: fertility, growth, prosperity, wealth, money, creativity, love, attraction, art, music, change and balance, Beltane, Yule, earth magic, compassion, heart chakra, Mother Earth, fairies, dryads, vegetation deities, the planet Venus, the element of earth, Venus, Cancer, Capricorn.

GREY: communication, study, teaching, divination, the planet Mercury.

INDIGO: perceptiveness, vision, intuition, insight, third eye chakra, Taurus.

MAGENTA: vision, creativity, insight, inspiration, creative vitality, root chakra.

ORANGE: optimism, success, courage, bravery, energy, ambition, luck, career, legal matters, self-esteem, spleen chakra, Samhain, Lughnasa, the sun, Leo.

PINK: love, romance, friendship, happiness, harmony, peace, compassion, handfastings, beauty, heart chakra, love goddesses, Libra.

PURPLE: strength, mastery, power, occult power, protection, Pisces, crone goddesses.

RED: life, vitality, energy, sex drive, passion, lust, conflict, competition, courage, strength, health, root chakra, Yule, Midsummer, fire spirits, mother goddesses, warrior gods, the planet Mars, the element of fire.

SILVER: intuition, truth, enlightenment, agriculture, the home, medicine, psychic ability, removes negativity, communication, personal enlightenment, moon rituals, moon goddesses.

TURQUOISE: inventiveness, conception, philosophy, creativity, communication, throat chakra.

VIOLET: spiritual healing, mastery, ceremony, spirituality, self-respect, spiritual growth, spiritual fulfilment, self-esteem, third eye chakra, crown chakra, Sagittarius.

WHITE: peace, cleansing, defensive magic, protection, purity, harmony, spirit, psychic development, the dispelling of negativity, purification, tranquillity, Imbolc, maiden goddesses, waxing moon, crown chakra.

YELLOW: intellectual development, strength of mind, learning, study, eloquence, joy, air spirits, vision, solar plexus chakra, the planet Mercury, the element of air, Ostara, the planet Mercury, Leo.

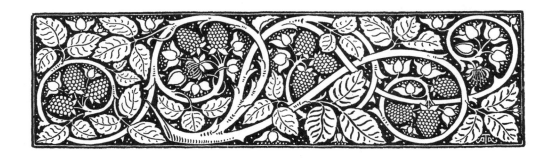

Herbs for Common Ailments

ARTHRITIS: basil, black pepper, cardamom, chilli, cinnamon, clove, coriander, fenugreek, ginger, lemon, oregano, parsley, rosemary, turmeric

ARTERIOSCLEROSIS: lemon

ATHLETE'S FOOT: garlic, thyme, turmeric

BAD BREATH: cardamom, clove, dill, peppermint, parsley

BLEPHARITIS: fennel

BLOATING: black pepper, caraway, cinnamon, coriander, dill, peppermint

BOILS, SKIN: caraway, garlic

BRONCHITIS: oregano, thyme

BRUISES: caraway, rosemary

BURSITIS: ginger, turmeric

CANDIDA ALBICANS: garlic

CANKERS: rosemary

CHEST CONGESTION, CATARRH: caraway, fennel, oregano

CHILBLAINS: garlic

CHOLESTEROL, HIGH: cinnamon, coriander, garlic, lemon, oats, turmeric

COLDS: black pepper, caraway, chilli, cinnamon, cumin, garlic, ginger, lemon, oregano, sage, thyme

CONJUNCTIVITIS: coriander, fennel

CONSTIPATION: cardamom, fenugreek

COUGHS: black pepper, cinnamon, clove, cumin, fennel, garlic, lemon, oregano, sage, thyme

CUTS: basil, cinnamon, thyme

CYSTITIS: lemon

DEPRESSION: basil, oregano

DERMATITIS: cardamom

DIARRHOEA: cinnamon, garlic, ginger

DYSPEPSIA: black pepper, caraway, cardamom, cinnamon, coriander, cumin, dill, fennel, ginger, lemon, peppermint, rosemary, thyme

EAR INFECTION: garlic

ECZEMA: basil, oats, sage, turmeric

FIBROMYALGIA: chilli

FLATULENCE: black pepper, caraway, cinnamon, coriander, dill, fennel, garlic, ginger, thyme

FLU: black pepper, chilli, ginger, peppermint, oregano, thyme

FUNGAL INFECTIONS: cardamom, oregano, thyme

GINGIVITIS: clove, thyme

GOUT: lemon, parsley

GUMS, INFLAMED: sage, thyme

HANGOVER: fennel, lemon, thyme

HEADACHE, SINUS: chilli

HEADACHE, TENSION: dill, rosemary, thyme

HEARTBURN: black pepper, fennel

HICCUPS: caraway, dill

HIGH BLOOD PRESSURE: cinnamon, garlic

IBS: cardamom, fennel, ginger, thyme

INDIGESTION: black pepper, caraway, cardamom, cinnamon, coriander, cumin, dill, fennel, ginger, lemon, peppermint, rosemary, thyme

INSECT BITES: garlic, peppermint, parsley, sage, thyme

INSOMNIA: basil, dill, oats

LARYNGITIS, HOARSENESS: caraway, fennel, fenugreek

MENOPAUSE: fennel, fenugreek, sage

MENSTRUAL CRAMPS: cinnamon, ginger

MIGRAINE: rosemary

MOTION SICKNESS: ginger

MUSCLE PAIN: black pepper, cardamom, chilli, cinnamon, clove, ginger, rosemary

MUSCLE SPASM: cardamom

NAUSEA: cinnamon, ginger, peppermint

OBESITY: black pepper, fennel

PERIODONTITIS: clove

PERIPHERAL NEUROPATHY: chilli

PSORIASIS: turmeric

RASHES: caraway, peppermint

RHEUMATISM: cardamom, coriander, fenugreek, lemon, oregano, parsley, rosemary

RINGWORM: garlic

ROSACEA: turmeric

SCLERODERMA: turmeric

SHINGLES: chilli

SORE THROAT: cardamom, fennel, fenugreek, peppermint, oregano, sage, thyme

SPRAINS: ginger, rosemary

STRESS: basil, peppermint

TENDONITIS: ginger

THRUSH, ORAL: basil, clove

THRUSH, VAGINAL: oregano

TONSILLITIS: sage

TOOTHACHE: clove, black pepper, peppermint

ULCER, MOUTH: cardamom, coriander, rosemary, sage, thyme

ULCERS, SKIN: basil

URINARY TRACT INFECTIONS: dill, garlic, parsley

VARICOSE VEINS: lemon

WARTS: garlic

WASP STING: lemon

WOUNDS, SMALL: basil, cinnamon, garlic, rosemary, sage, thyme, turmeric

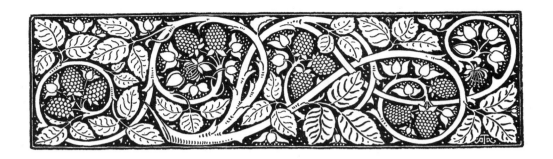

Glossary of Herbal Terminology

ABORTIFACIENT: induces abortion

ADAPTOGENS: herbs that help us adapt to stress by supporting the adrenal glands, the endocrine system, and the whole person. These herbs help us adapt to stress by supporting the adrenal glands, the endocrine system. They work holistically.

ADJUVANT: aids the action of a medicinal agent

ALTERATIVE: herbs alter or change a long-standing condition by aiding the elimination of metabolic toxins. Known as "blood cleansers" in the past, these herbs improve lymphatic circulation, boost immunity, and help clear chronic conditions, particularly of the skin. These herbs help chronic conditions because they aid in the elimination of metabolic toxins.

AMOEBICIDAL: treats diseases caused by amoeba such as amoebic dysentery

ANAESTHETICS: induces loss of sensation or consciousness due to the depression of nerve function

ANALEPTIC: restorative or stimulating effect on central nervous system

ANALGESIC: relieves pain

ANAPHRODISIAC: decreases sexual desires

ANODYNE: relieves pain

ANTACID: neutralises excess acid produced by the stomach

ANTHELMINTIC: an agent that destroys and expels worms from the intestines

ANTIANAEMIC: prevents or cures anaemia

ANTIBACTERIAL: destroys or stops the growth of bacteria

ANTIBILIOUS: combats nausea

ANTIBIOTIC: inhibits the growth of germs, bacteria, and harmful microbes

ANTICATARRH: reduces inflamed mucous membranes of head and throat

ANTIDEPRESSANT: therapy that acts to prevent, cure, or alleviate mental depression

ANTIDIABETIC: lowers blood sugar

ANTIDIARRHOEAL: substances used to prevent or treat diarrhoea

ANTIEMETIC: stops vomiting

ANTIEPILEPTIC: combats the convulsions or seizures of epilepsy

ANTIFUNGAL: destroys or inhibits the growth of fungus

ANTIHEAMORRHAGIC: controls haemorrhaging or bleeding

ANTI-INFECTIOUS: counteracts infection

ANTI-INFLAMMATORY: controls inflammation, a reaction to injury or infection

ANTILITHIC: combats the formation of stones in the kidneys and bladder

ANTIMALARIAL: preventing or relieving malaria

ANTIMICROBIAL: destructive to microbes

ANTIOXIDANT: prevents or inhibits oxidation

ANTIPERIODIC: prevents the periodic recurrence of attacks of a disease

ANTIPHLOGISTIC: counteracts inflammation.

ANTIPRURITIC: prevents or relieves itching

ANTIPYRETIC: agent that reduces fever (febrifuge)

ANTIPYRETIC: reduces fever

ANTIRHEUMATIC: eases pain of rheumatism, inflammation of joints and muscles

ANTISCORBUTIC: prevents or treats scurvy

ANTISEPTIC: prevents decay or putrefaction

ANTISPASMODIC: relieves or prevents involuntary muscle spasms or cramps

ANTITUSSIVE: controls or prevents cough

ANTIVENOMOUS: acts against poisonous matter from animals

ANTIVIRAL: opposes the action of a virus

ANTIZYMOTIC: herbs that destroy disease-producing organisms

APERIENT: a very mild laxative

APERITIVE: stimulates the appetite for food

APHRODISIAC: a substance that increases capacity for sexual arousal

APPETIZER: stimulates the appetite

AROMATIC: a herb with a pleasant, fragrant scent and a pungent taste

ASEPSIS: sterile, a condition free of germs, infection, and any form of life

ASTRINGENT: causes a local contraction of the skin, blood vessels, and other tissues, thereby arresting the discharge of blood, mucus, etc.

BALSAMIC: a healing or soothing agent

BITTER: stimulates appetite or digestive function

CALMATIVE: herbs that are soothing or sedating

CARDIAC STIMULANT: herbs that promote circulation when there is a weak heart

CARDIOTONIC: increases strength and tone (normal tension or response to stimuli) of the heart

CARMINATIVE: causes the release of stomach or intestinal gas

CATARRHAL: pertains to inflammation of mucous membranes of the head and throat

CATHARTIC: an active purgative, producing bowel movements

CHOLAGOGUE: increases flow of bile from gallbladder

CICATRIZANT: aids formation of scar tissue and healing wounds

COUNTERIRRITANT: produces an inflammatory response for affecting an adjacent area

DECONGESTANT: relieves congestion

DEMULCENT: soothing action on an inflammation

DEPURATIVE: purifies and cleanses the blood

DETERGENT: cleanses boils, ulcers, wounds, etc.

DIAPHORETIC: promotes perspiration

DIGESTIVES: assists the stomach and intestines in normal digestion

DISCUTIENT: dissolves or causes something, such as a tumour, to disappear

DISINFECTANT: destroys germs

DIURETIC: increases urine flow

DRASTIC: violent purgative

ECBOLIC: increases contractions of uterus, facilitating childbirth

EMETIC: causes vomiting

EMMENAGOGUE: brings on menstruation

EMOLLIENT: softens and soothes the skin

EPISPASTIC: locally applied to the skin

ERRHINE: brings on sneezing, increasing flow of mucus in nasal passages

ESCHAROTIC: a caustic substance that destroys tissue and causes sloughing

ESCULENT: edible

EUPHORIANT: produces a sense of bodily comfort—a temporary, often addictive effect

EXANTHEMATOUS: remedy for skin eruptions such as measles, etc.

EXHILARANT: enlivens and cheers the mind

EXPECTORANT: promotes the ejection of mucus or exudate from the lungs, bronchi, and trachea

FEBRIFUGE: reduces or relieves a fever

GALACTOGOGUE: increases breast milk secretion

GERMICIDE: destroys germs and worms

GERMIFUGE: expels germs

HEMAGOGUE: an agent that promotes the flow of blood

HEMOSTATIC: controls the flow or stops the flow of blood

HEPATIC: having to do with the liver

HYPERTENSIVE: raises blood pressure

HYPNOTIC: induces sleep

HYPOGLYCEMANT: lowers blood sugar

HYPOTENSIVE: lowers blood pressure

LACTIFUGE: reduces the flow of breast milk

LAXATIVE: acts to loosen the bowels' contents

LITHOTRIPTIC: causes dissolution or destruction of stones in the bladder or kidneys

MASTICATORY: increases flow of saliva upon chewing

MATURATING: promotes the bringing to a head of boils, etc.

MUCILAGINOUS: has a soothing effect on inflamed mucous membranes

NARCOTIC: induces drowsiness and lessens pain

NAUSEANT: causes nausea and vomiting

NERVINE: nerve tonic

OESTROGENIC: causes the production of oestrogen

OPTHALMICUM: remedy for diseases of the eye

PARASITICIDE: destroys parasites

PARTURIENT/PARTURIFACIANT: induces childbirth or labour

PUNGENT: a sharp sensation of taste or smell

PURGATIVE: promotes the vigorous evacuation of the bowels

REFRIGERANT: lowers body temperature

RELAXANT: relieves tension, especially muscular tension

RESORBENT: aids reabsorption of blood from bruises

RUBEFACIENT: reddens the skin by increasing the local blood supply

SEDATIVE: has tranquilizing effect on the body

SIALAGOGUE: promotes the flow of saliva

SOPORIFIC: induces sleep

STIMULANT: temporarily increases body or organ function

STOMACHIC: aids the stomach and digestion action

STYPTIC: causes vascular contraction of the blood vessels to arrest haemorrhage and bleeding

SUDORIFIC: increases perspiration

TONIC: increases strength and tone

VERMICIDE: kills intestinal worms

VERMIFUGE: expels intestinal worms or parasites

VESICANT: causes blistering

VULNERARY: used in treating fresh cuts and wounds

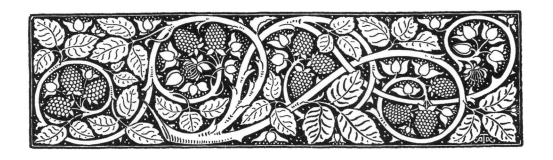

Cosmetic Uses of Herbs in This Book

ACNE: black pepper, clove, fennel, garlic, lemon, oregano, rosemary, thyme, turmeric

AGE SPOTS (LIVER SPOTS): cumin, lemon, parsley

ANTIBACTERIAL: basil, black pepper, cardamom, cinnamon, fenugreek, lemon, oregano, parsley, thyme, turmeric

ANTIFUNGAL: cardamom, oregano

ANTI-INFLAMMATORY: cardamom, fenugreek, oats, turmeric

ANTIOXIDANT: basil, caraway, cinnamon, coriander, cumin, ginger, oregano, parsley

ASTRINGENT: lemon, rosemary, sage, thyme

BLEMISHES AND PIMPLES: lemon, oregano, rosemary, thyme, turmeric

CELLULITE: fennel, garlic

COLLAGEN STIMULATANT: cinnamon, turmeric

DANDRUFF: cardamom, fennel, garlic, lemon, rosemary, thyme

DEODORANT: mint, sage

EXFOLIATING: black pepper, fennel, fenugreek, mint

EYES, PUFFY: fennel, parsley

HAIR LOSS: garlic, rosemary

HAIR, DARKEN: sage

HAIR, FRIZZY: mint

HAIR, LIGHTEN: lemon

HAIR, OILY: lemon

HAIR, SHINE: fenugreek, mint, rosemary, sage

HAIR, STIMULATE: cardamom, cinnamon, fenugreek, garlic, rosemary, thyme

PORES, ENLARGED: fennel

SCALP, DRY: cardamom

SCALP, IRRITATED: cardamom, fennel, oregano

SKIN TONE, EVEN: basil, garlic, parsley, turmeric

SKIN, DULL: lemon, oats, parsley

SKIN, OILY: lemon, mint, thyme

SKIN, PLUMP UP: cinnamon

SKIN, REJUVENATE: basil, fenugreek, lemon, oats, rosemary, turmeric

SKIN, REPAIR: fenugreek

SKIN, ROUGH: lemon

SKIN, SOFTEN: fennel, fenugreek, lemon, mint

SKIN, STIMULATE CIRCULATION: garlic, turmeric

SKIN, TIGHTEN: basil, cinnamon, coriander, cumin, dill, fennel, garlic, oats, thyme

TEETH, WHITEN: sage

WRINKLES: coriander, fennel, fenugreek, lemon, oats, turmeric

• • • • •

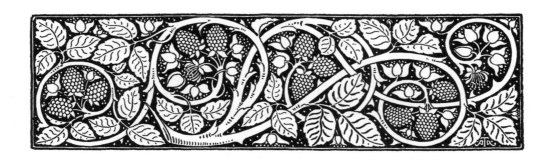

Weights and Measures

Volume
(Liquid Measures)

METRIC	US CUPS
15 MILLILITRES	1 TABLESPOON
30 MILLILITRES	2 TABLESPOONS
60 MILLILITRES	¼ CUP
75 MILLILITRES	⅓ CUP
120 MILLILITRES	½ CUP
150 MILLILITRES	⅔ CUP
180 MILLILITRES	¾ CUP
250 MILLILITRES	1 CUP
310 MILLILITRES	1¼ CUPS
620 MILLILITRES	2½ CUPS

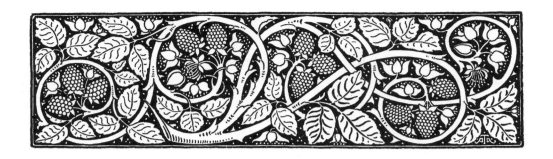

Select Bibliography

Bartram, Thomas. *Bartram's Encyclopaedia of Herbal Medicine*. London: Constable and Robinson, 1998.

Beyerl, Paul. *The Master Book of Herbalism*. Washington: Phoenix Publishing, 1984.

Bingen, Hildegard von. *Causae et Curae*. Translated by Manfred Pawlik and Patrick Madigan. Collegeville, MN: Liturgical Press, 1994.

Boxer, Arabella, and Philippa Back. *The Herb Book*. London: Octopus Books, 1980.

Bremness, Lesley. *The Complete Book of Herbs: A Practical Guide to Growing and Using Herbs*. New York: Viking, 1994.

Brown, Deni. *Encyclopedia of Herbs and Their Uses*. New York: Dorling Kindersley, 1995.

Brunton-Seal, Julie, and Matthew Seal. *Kitchen Medicine*. London: Merlin Unwin Books, 2010.

Buhner, Stephen Harrod. *Sacred and Herbal Healing Beers*. Boulder, CO: Siris Books, 1998.

Burr Thompson, Dorothy, and Ralph E. Griswold. *Garden Lore of Ancient Athens*. Princeton, NJ: American School of Classical Studies at Athens, 1963.

Castleman, Michael. *The Healing Herbs*. Emmaus, PA: Rodale Press, 1991.

———. *The New Healing Herbs*. New York: Rodale, 2001.

Chevalier, Andrew. *The Encyclopaedia of Medicinal Plants*. London: Dorling Kindersley, 1996.

Chown, Vicky, and Kim Walker. *The Handmade Apothecary*. London: Kyle Books, 2017.

Culpeper, Nicholas. *Culpeper's Complete Herbal*. London: W. Foulsham and Co.

D'Andréa, Jeanne. *Ancient Herbs in the J. Paul Getty Museum Gardens*. New York: The J. Paul Getty Museum, 1982.

Down, Deni. *The Royal Horticultural Society Encyclopaedia of Herbs and Their Uses*. London: Dorling Kindersley, 1997.

Easley, Thomas, and Steven Horne. *The Modern Herbal Dispensatory*. Berkeley, CA: North Atlantic Books, 2016.

Edwards, Gail Faith. *Opening Our Wild Hearts to the Healing Herbs*. Woodstock, NY: Ash Tree Publishing, 2000.

Elworthy, Frederick Thomas. *The Evil Eye: An Account of This Ancient and Widespread Superstition*. London: John Murray, 1895.

Farrar, Linda. *Gardens and Gardeners of the Ancient World: History, Myth and Archaeology*. Windgather Press, 2016.

Folkard, Richard. *Plant Lore, Legends, and Lyrics: Embracing the Myths, Traditions, Superstitions, and Folk-Lore of the Plant Kingdom*. CreateSpace Independent Publishing Platform, 2017.

Franklin, Anna, and Sue Lavender. *Herb Craft*. Chieveley: Capall Bann, 1995.

Franklin, Anna. *Hearth Witch*. Earl Shilton: Lear Books, 2004.

————. *Working with Fairies*. Career Press, 2006.

Gahlin, Lucia. *Gods and Myths of Ancient Egypt*. Southwater, 2014.

Genders, Roy. *Natural Beauty*. Lucerne: EMB Services, 1992.

Gerard, John. *Gerard's Herbal*. London: Senate, 1994.

Gladstar, Rosemary. *Family Herbal*. North Adams, MA: Storey Publishing, 2001.

Goff, Barbara. *Citizen Bacchae: Women's Ritual Practice in Ancient Greece*. University of California Press, 2004.

Gordon, Lesley. *A Country Herbal*. London: Peerage Books, 1980.

Green, James. *The Herbal Medicine Maker's Handbook*. Berkeley: Crossing Press, 2002.

Green, M. *Gods of the Celts*. Gloucester: Allan Sutton, 1986.

Grieve, Mrs. M. *A Modern Herbal*. London: Johnathon Cape, 1931. New York: Dover, 1981.

Griggs, Barbara. *Green Pharmacy: A History of Herbal Medicine*. New York: Viking Press, 1982.

· · · · ·

Guyton, Anita. *The Book of Natural Beauty*. London: Stanley Paul and Co. Ltd., 1981.

Hemphill, Rosemary. *Herbs for All Seasons*. London: Penguin, 1975.

Herodotus. *The History of Herodotus*. Translated by G. C. Macaulay. London: Macmillan, 1890.

Hesiod. Theogony. Online at http://www.perseus.tufts.edu/hopper /text?doc=Perseus%3Atext%3A1999.01.0130%3Acard%3D1 (accessed 14 December 2017).

Hoffman, David. *The Holistic Herbal*. Shaftsbury: Element Books, 1986.

———. *Medical Herbalism*. Rochester: Healing Arts Press, 2003.

Holmes, Peter. *The Energetics of Western Herbs*. Boulder, CO: Artemis Press, 1989.

Homer. *The Odyssey*. Translated by E. V. Rieu. New York: Penguin Classics, 2003.

Knapp, Stephen. *Krishna Deities and Their Miracles*. Prabhat Prakashan, 2011.

Levy, Isaac Jack, and Rosemary Levy Zumwalt. *Ritual Medical Lore of Sephardic Women: Sweetening the Spirits, Healing the Sick*. University of Illinois Press, 2002.

Little, Kitty. *Kitty Little's Book of Herbal Beauty*. Harmondsworth: Penguin Books, 1981.

Lust, John. *The Herb Book*. Bantam Books, 1974.

Mabey, Richard. *Flora Britannica*. London: Sinclair-Stevenson, 1996.

Moore, A. W. *The Folk-Lore of the Isle of Man*. London: D. Nutt, 1891.

Nilsson, Martin P. *Greek Popular Religion*. New York: Columbia University Press, 1940.

Ody, Penelope. *The Complete Medicinal Herbal*. London: Dorling Kindersley, 1993.

Passebecq, Andre. *Aromatherapy*. Wellingborough: Thorsons, 1979.

Peter, Holmes. *The Energetics of Western Herbs*. Boulder, CO: Snow Lotus Press, 1997.

Petropoulos, John, ed. *Greek Magic: Ancient, Medieval and Modern*. Routledge, 2008.

Pliny the Elder. *The Natural History*. Translated by H. Rackham. Loeb Classical Library 370, 1945.

Power, Henry and Leonard William Sedgwick. *The New Sydenham Society's Lexicon of Medicine and the Allied Sciences (Based on Mayne's Lexicon)*. New Sydenham Society, 1881.

Pughe, John, translator. *The Physicians of Myddfai*. Felinach: The Welsh Mss. Society, facsimile reprint Llanerch Publishers, 1993.

Rätsch, Christian, and Claudia Müller-Ebeling. *The Encyclopedia of Aphrodisiacs: Psychoactive Substances for Use in Sexual Practices*. Park Street Press, 2013.

· · · · ·

Raven, J. E. *Plants and Plant Lore in Ancient Greece*. Oxford: Leopard's Head Press, 2000.

Sarton, George. *Introduction to the History of Science. vol. 1: From Homer to Omar Khayyam.* Baltimore, MD: William and Wilkins, 1927.

Segal, Charles. *Dionysiac Poetics and Euripides' Bacchae*. Princeton University Press, 1997.

Sesha, T. R. Iyengar. *Dravidian India*. Asian Educational Services, 2000.

Sharma, Mahesh. *Western Himalayan Temple Records: State, Pilgrimage, Ritual and Legality in Chamba*. Brill, 2009.

Simoons, Frederick J. *Plants of Life, Plants of Death*. The University of Wisconsin Press, 1998.

Smith, Frederick M. *The Self Possessed: Deity and Spirit Possession in South Asian Literature and Civilization*. Columbia University Press, 2012.

Stapley, Christina. *Herbcraft Naturally*. Chichester: Heartsease Books, 1994.

Steel, Susannah, editor. *Healing Foods: Neal's Yard Remedies*. London: Dorling Kindersley, 2013.

———. *Neal's Yard Remedies*. London: Dorling Kindersley, 2010.

Strabo, Walafrid. *On the Cultivation of Gardens*. Translated by James Mitchell. San Francisco: Ithuriel's Spear, 2008.

Strabo. *The Geographica*. Translated by H. C. Hamilton and W. Falconer, 1903. Online at http://www.perseus.tufts.edu/hopper/

Swain, J. O. *The Lore of Spices*. London: Grange Books, 1991.

Theophrastus. *Enquiry Into Plants*, volume 1: books 1–5. Translated by Arthur F. Hort. Loeb Classical Library 70, 1916.

Vickery, Roy. *Oxford Dictionary of Plant Lore*. Oxford: Oxford UP, 1995.

Virgil. *Eclogues. Georgics. Aenid:* books 1–6. Translated by H. Rushton Fairclough. Loeb Classical Library, revised edition. Harvard UP, 1999.

Watts, D. C. *Elsevier's Dictionary of Plant Lore*. London: Academic Press, 2007.

Weed, Susun S. *Healing Wise*. Woodstock, NY: Ash Tree Publishing, 1989.

Wong, James. *Grow Your Own Drugs*. London: HarperCollins, 2009.

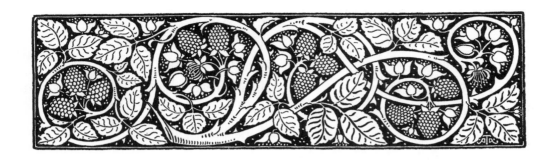

Recipe Index

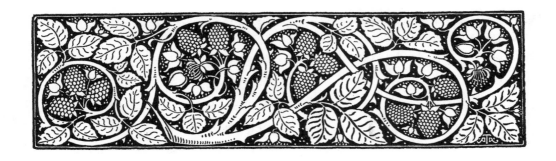

Index

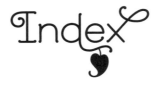